W9-CSX-207

Taking Charge of Your Child's Allergies

The Informed Parent's Comprehensive Guide

This book is for our wives, Laurel and Jean, mothers who have dealt each day with their own children's allegies with incomparable understanding and patience.

Taking Charge of Your Child's Allergies

The Informed Parent's Comprehensive Guide

M. Eric Gershwin, MD
University of California Medical School, Davis, CA

Edwin L. Klingelhofer, PhD
Professor Emeritus of Psychology
California State University, Sacramento, CA

Humana Press ✳ Totowa, New Jersey

© 1998 Humana Press Inc.
999 Riverview Drive, Suite 208
Totowa, New Jersey 07512

For additional copies, pricing for bulk purchases, and/or information about other Humana titles, contact Humana at the above address or at any of the following numbers: Tel: 973-256-1699; Fax: 973-256-8341; E-mail: humana@humanapr.com, or visit our Website: http://humanapr.com

This publication is printed on acid-free paper. ∞
ANSI Z39.48-1984 (American National Standards Institute) Permanence of Paper for Printed Library Materials.

Cover and template designs by Patricia F. Cleary.

Photocopy Authorization Policy:
Authorization to photocopy items for internal or personal use, or the internal or personal use of specific clients, is granted by Humana Press Inc., provided that the base fee of US $8.00 per copy, plus US $00.25 per page, is paid directly to the Copyright Clearance Center at 222 Rosewood Drive, Danvers, MA 01923. For those organizations that have been granted a photocopy license from the CCC, a separate system of payment has been arranged and is acceptable to Humana Press Inc. The fee code for users of the Transactional Reporting Service is: [0-89603-455-0/98 $8.00 + $00.25].

Printed in the United States of America. 10 9 8 7 6 5 4 3 2 1

Library of Congress Cataloging in Publication Data

Gershwin, M. Eric

    Taking charge of your child's allergies: the informed parent's comprehensive guide / M. Eric Gershwin, Edwin L. Klingelhofer.
       p. cm.
    Includes index.
    ISBN 0-89603-455-0 (alk. paper)
    1. Allergy in children—Popular works. 2. Allergy in children—Patients—Care. 3. Allergy in children—Prevention. 4. Parent and child. 5. Consumer education. I. Klingelhofer, E. L. (Ed L.) II. Title.
    RJ386.G465   1998   98-5850
    618.92'97—dc21   CIP

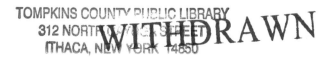

Preface

The number of children with allergies is astounding—nearly one child in six is said to suffer from some sort of allergy. The problems of these allergic children can be as mild as occasional attacks of hay fever or as severe as disfiguring eczema and life-threatening bronchial asthma. In addition to the obvious health problems associated with having allergies, affected children may experience recurring colds, painful ear infections, and other allergy-linked conditions, all of which cause frequent school absences. Childhood allergies affect school performance adversely; they may be instrumental in reducing attention span, and they are certainly a major social, psychological, and financial burden for children and their parents.

This book is a complete guide to childhood allergies presented in simple jargon-free language. It provides parents with comprehensive, up-to-date, and practical information and advice on how to help their allergic children. It identifies the many allergic symptoms, tells what they look like, how prevalent they are, what causes them, and what to do about them. It outlines steps parents can take to help their children understand, manage, and control their allergies. Its goal is to help parents and children cope effectively with a major childhood problem.

We wrote this book because we have had to live with allergies all our lives, in ourselves and in our children. Both of us have had severely allergic children. We want to share with you what we have found out, and what Eric, who is a Professor of Medicine and Chief of Allergy, Rheumatology, and Clinical Immunology at the University of California, Davis, Medical School, teaches his medical students about caring for allergic children.

M. Eric Gershwin
Edwin L. Klingelhofer

To Our Readers

This book can help you and your family greatly. Its suggestions about health care reflect the best and most up-to-date medical information and opinions available. As with all medical advice, however, cases—and treatments thereof—may vary.

The authors and publisher therefore disclaim any responsibility for consequences resulting from following advice or procedures set forth in this book. It is not intended to be an alternative to or substitute for your own doctor's recommendations. In particular, the treatment of severe, protracted, or stubborn symptoms or the use of any drug or medication should be undertaken only after consultation with your own physician.

Contents

PART II. WHAT ARE ALLERGIES' TRIGGERS AND HOW CAN I AVOID OR CONTROL THEM EFFECTIVELY?

Chapter 4. Food and Food Additives

Chapter 5. Colds and Respiratory Infections

Chapter 6. Airborne Allergens

Chapter 7. Weather, Climate, and Exercise

Introduction

Technological change has left no aspect of life in the United States untouched. Health care has been dramatically affected by these developments; complex and exquisitely delicate treatments and procedures, unimaginable fifty years ago, are now routine. Common childhood diseases have been all but eradicated and an arsenal of drugs and antibiotics that directly attack the causes of illness have been brought into general use. Along with these improvements in technique and medication, improved understanding of the interplay of nutrition, activity, and physical well-being have helped to prolong and improve the overall quality of life.

The ability to understand and care for allergies is one area that has benefited mightily from this explosion of knowledge. Unearthing the mechanisms that trigger allergies, discovering medications that effectively relieve allergic symptoms, and developing potent coping strategies have served to render allergies more manageable and less debilitating than they have ever been. Yet, as these developments have taken place, the incidence of allergies has increased markedly and some forms of allergic disease have become especially virulent.

Allergies are among the most common and troublesome ailments around. Childhood allergies are so widespread that nearly half of all American families can point to at least one member who is troubled with one form or another of allergic disease. The rising incidence owes something to the greatly improved ability to identify symptoms as allergic, but environmental degradation doubtless sets off reactions that would not have manifested themselves in less toxic times.

The growing prevalence of allergies, especially among children, their increasing severity, and the need for parents to be able to make informed, effective decisions about the care and treatment of their allergic offspring are factors that have led us to write this book. Allergic children need smart, timely care; without it, severe hard-to-manage conditions may result. All too often we see allergic children needlessly troubled with problems, sometimes severe, that grow out of inappropriate or bungled treatment—poor appetite, sleep disturbance, attention disorder, irritability, anxiety, even depression.

> Bill, now in high school, had been troubled by recurrent colds, sore throats, and ear infections from the time he was a toddler. His grades in school were consistently below average and he displayed little interest in his school work. His parents felt that their home away from home was the doctor's office, mainly because of Bill's recurring and excruciatingly painful earaches. Bill's father had always wondered about the bluish discoloration under his son's eyes and happened to mention them to a physician he saw when taking an insurance physical. The doctor suggested that Bill's eye discoloration might be a condition called "shiners" and that he could be suffering from allergies. The parents took Bill to an allergist who established that Bill was severely allergic to house dust. The dust allergy had caused chronic irritation of nasal membranes, blockage of the eustachian tube, and the frequent infection-caused earaches. Acting on the allergist's advice, Bill's parents installed an air cleaner and took drastic measures to render their home and car as free of dust as possible. The results were immensely gratifying. Not only did the earaches stop but, in a matter of months, Bill's school performance improved to the point where he earned a place on the honor roll and became a serious, motivated student interested in and enjoying school and school activities.

The point is that the family doctor should have recognized the tell-tale symptoms years before the correct diagnosis was finally made and the parents, for their part, should have looked for help elsewhere when Bill's condition persisted.

The questions parents ask (and that are the focus of this book) are:
- How should we go about looking after an allergic child?
- How can we be sure that our child's problems are really due to allergies?
- What are the tell-tale signs we should know about in caring for our allergic child?
- Do allergic diseases have any special features that we need to be alert to?
- How are allergies treated? What can be done to manage them better or eliminate them altogether?
- Do all doctors treat allergies in the same way? How do we find a doctor who will help us deal effectively with our child's allergies?
- What can we do to assist our allergic child–and all of the other members of he family, including ourselves to lead a normal life?

The goal of this book is to help you answer these questions. You will see that it is very different from other books on allergy. Though the information and suggestions it contains are up-to-the-minute and medically proven, its language is simple and free as we could make it of medical terms or highly technical explanations. Charts to help you decide, step-by-step, what you should do about specific signs and symptoms you see in you child appear throughout. Above all, it strives to show you how you can take greater responsibility for the knowledgeable, effective, aggressive management of your child's symptoms. This skillful management can minimize or totally eliminate the possible life-long negative effects that can be the unwanted result of neglected or poorly treated allergies.

The book has five major divisions. Part I offers a general introduction to childhood allergies—what they are, who has them, what effects they have, and what can be done about them. Part II names and discusses in detail the major triggers of allergies and what measures can be used to mitigate their effects, while each of Part III's chapters deal with a specific allergic disease and spells out what you can do to diagnose, treat, control, and avoid symptoms of the complaint.

Part IV examines the role that allergies may play in relation to the general health problems all children experience, and how the general problems may interact with or abet allergic tendencies.

Part V spells out detailed steps and strategies you can follow to provide your child with an environment that is as free as possible of the antigens— allergy causing substances—and irritants that are the root cause of so many symptoms. It also offers advice that cover things you need to know to make informed decisions about care for your allergic child, from understanding and dealing with AIDS, to suggestions about how to locate and choose a physician, to discussions of vaccinations and the appropriateness of allergy shots.

Finally, we include a series of Appendices to provide useful current information about sources of triggers, as well as discussions of and recommendations regarding special diets.

Though we do our best to say all that needs to be said about treatment, our primary emphasis throughout is on prevention. It is far easier—and far, far less costly—to prevent allergic symptoms than to treat them once they appear. Being able to recognize tell-tale-signs early on, and being able to diagnose and then learn to follow preventive or avoidance tactics unfailingly are the keys to the successful management of all but the most severe and chronic conditions.

You, as parent of an allergic child, will need to make complex difficult decisions. The bottom line is that if you make them properly, knowledgeably, and with the right kind of help, your child will in turn be helped immeasurably. Much of that help is to be found in these pages.

Part One

What Are Allergies,

Why Do Children Have Them,

How Can I Be Sure My Child
Is Really Allergic,
And How Best Can I Cope?

1

Why Our Child?

The initial shock when parents learn their child is allergic can be distressing. Parents invariably want to know: "Why our child?" "Will our other children come down with the same thing?" "Will it develop into asthma?" They then eye each other, either in the doctor's office or back home, and wonder if the partner or their own self is somehow at fault.

Some Facts About Allergies

Allergies, though commonplace, are not very well understood; there is probably more misinformation about allergies around than there is solid fact. One stubborn bit of misinformation is the myth that allergies are psychologically caused—"All in the head," as the saying goes—with the parents somehow bearing the blame for the child's sickness. When the parents ask, "Why Janie?" they really want to know, "What have we done to cause this suffering; what is wrong with our parenting, our cooking, whatever—and what can we do to fix things?" They also want to know where the disease originated—whose family passed it along to the child.

Allergies, despite the misinformation and mystery that shroud them, are straightforward medical problems, not psychologically caused, and not the outgrowth of parental incompetence or neglect. And they are epidemic. Rare is the family completely free of allergic problems. Thus, if your child suffers from an allergy, he or she does not suffer alone. More than 50 million Americans, adults and children, have allergies. No population group anywhere in the world is allergy-free, although there are striking differences in the incidence and severity of allergies among them. In West Africa and among Native Americans, asthma is quite rare, but one in three inhabitants of the British West Indies has it.

In this country, rural residents, probably because they run into more of the triggers (allergens) than city dwellers, are more prone to have hay fever;

some ethnic groups, notably African-Americans, show higher incidences of allergic diseases. Urban dwellers, particularly children in inner cities, have a phenomenal rate and severity of asthma; the degradation of our environment, especially the air we breathe, is associated with a 100% increase in the prevalence of asthma since 1979. Twenty-one percent of all deaths attributed to asthma, in the 16–25 age range, in the United States, occur in Chicago and New York City alone.

The tendency to develop allergies is inherited or hereditary, but environmental or acquired factors play a role. The hereditary basis has been established in several ways. Depending on the specific allergic complaint, a child whose parents have the condition is anywhere from two to five times more likely to turn up with the problem than a child whose parents are free of symptoms. Other investigations have shown that if one member of a pair of identical twins has an allergy, the other twin will almost certainly develop it, although nonidentical twins, even though they share the same environment, are not nearly as likely to share the same allergy.

Whether or not an allergy develops in your child depends, in the final analysis, on being exposed to its cause. If your child is genetically disposed to develop an allergic reaction to penicillin, he or she will develop this reaction only if penicillin is administered. Even if there is inherited sensitivity to ragweed, a French child would not develop ragweed-caused hay fever simply because France is ragweed-free. However, if the family emigrated to Michigan the child would show hay fever symptoms within a few years.

Also, unhappily, in children allergies can have much more serious physical and social consequences than they do in adults. Consider:

- Asthma is much more prevalent and severe—in some instances life-threatening—in children.
- Eczema, an extremely uncomfortable and hard-to-manage complaint, commonly starts in early childhood.
- Nasal allergies trigger serious, recurring ear infections and chronic headaches in many youngsters.
- Allergy medications—especially those used to treat asthma—can be disagreeable to take and carry anything from unpleasant to dangerous side effects. Children often resist taking them, but, when used properly, they can be wonderfully beneficial.
- Allergies are often responsible for extended and frequent school absences and poor school performance.
- Chronic allergies can have diffuse and troublesome psychological consequences, impairing normal development and adjustment and causing great difficulty and handicaps in later life.

- Unless you, as a care provider, are prepared, your chronically allergic child can play havoc with your and other family members' lives. Care for an ailing child, which can be expensive and time-, energy-, and attention-consuming, may override all other considerations, and disrupt normal family activities and interrelationships.

These problems are also exacerbated by the characteristics of the children as they pass through the several developmental stages. During *infancy*, parents sense that something is the matter, but because of the inability of the child to communicate, have no idea of the nature of the trouble.

In *early childhood*, the ability to communicate improves, but it may be accompanied by confusion, little or no comprehension of what is happening, and the formation of stubborn or irrational fears of or aversions to treatment, especially when it comes to taking unpleasant-tasting medicines or having shots.

In *later childhood and adolescence*, self-knowledge (and knowledge of personal strengths and weaknesses) grows and, with this, some sense of how to manage the complaint, whatever it is. The bad news is that at this stage the need to be like other children intensifies and, with it, a strong tendency to resist avoidance or treatment measures intended to manage the allergy. All too often adolescents seem to prefer risking illness to being seen as different or conspicuous by taking steps to avoid pollens or publicly using an asthma inhaler during an attack.

Penny, 14, hates being an asthmatic and goes to painful lengths to conceal her condition from her peers. She believes being seen using her Ventolin™ inhaler would give away her secret so she takes great care never to use it in public. She has also been told to use a peak flow meter regularly to monitor her condition, but does not even know where the device is. What happens, though, is that she does have episodes of wheezing in class that soon intensify to the point where everyone in the room hears and is troubled by her coughing and wheezing. Her asthma is the worst-kept secret in the high school.

It will help you, at all points, to learn as much as you can about the condition, its cause, treatment, consequences, and how it is linked to other childhood illnesses, allergic and otherwise. This search for causes and relationships will help you and your child cope with the problem and steer clear of hazards down the road.

Eczema, for example, most often turns up in infants. It is a distressing but easily treatable complaint that, if addressed promptly and competently, will leave no psychological or physical scars. It is likely to be followed by other allergic problems in childhood—asthma and hay fever particularly—and the informed parent will know what steps to take if these conditions do turn up. By recognizing these possibilities, many of the tribulations associated with allergies, such as visits to a series of specialists, conflicting diagnoses, and the attendant confusion, expense, and school absence can often be circumvented. Good parents, good drivers, and good ball players have this in common—they know in advance what they will do when a given event happens, and they are prepared to do it the moment it develops.

> Jason has had eczema from the time he was 6 months old. His mother has meticulously avoided using soaps, and she keeps his skin as moist and as lubricated as possible. Jason is now 11 years old, and for the past 3 or 4 weeks his eczema has clearly gotten worse. His mother is perplexed concerning what is happening. She is convinced she is doing everything right, but missing a clue. She even goes so far as to track and follow Jason throughout the day. After 4 days, she can find nothing whatsoever to point to the source of the trouble, so she speaks to the pediatrician. He asks her about her laundry detergent. Jason's mom says that she has been using only about one-fourth the recommended amount of laundry detergent on Jason's clothes and has not changed her method of washing in many years. However, the question about detergent reminds her that she has recently started using a fabric softener. (She thought the fabric softener would soften Jason's clothes and make them less harsh to his skin.) She has completely forgotten this change in routine because she started the fabric softener some 2 months before Jason's skin began to worsen. Jason's doctor has not heard that fabric softener triggers eczema, but advises her to discontinue using it. Within 2 weeks of stopping the fabric softener, Jason's skin returns to its earlier state—readily managed mild eczema.

Parents with allergic children have the additional burden of learning and adhering conscientiously to treatment procedures for their child's complaint; they should know how to avoid and control exposure to triggers that cause allergies to develop; they should encourage and assist the child in pursuing as close to a full, normal, autonomous life as possible, given the allergy, and they should continually remind themselves that:

- At some time or another, allergies turn up in most families.
- Allergies and asthma are not psychologically or emotionally caused.
- It is not the child's fault that he or she is allergic. Inner force, strength of character, or high resolve will not make the allergy vanish.
- Correct medications, properly taken, will usually improve, but will not "cure" allergies.

However, on the up side:

- You cannot catch an allergy from someone else.
- Most allergies do become better as children grow older; happily, their physiology changes and they become easier to treat.
- Properly watched and prepared, allergic children can do most everything other children do, including taking part in physical edu-

cation in school, attending summer camp, and competing in serious, even (given the talent) world-class athletics.

- Allergies need not and can be kept from dragging down school academic performance or interfering with the joy and excitement of growing up.
- Effective management of allergies in children is possible with sensible, informed, perceptive, alert, conscientious parents.

What Specifically Is an Allergy?

An allergy is a special and unique response by your body to a foreign substance. Your body senses that it has inhaled, swallowed, or touched something foreign and it responds to this intruder by making an antibody called immunoglobulin E (IgE). Most often this response is to substances we inhale, like pollen, dust, or animal dander, or things we swallow, like food. Our environment contains millions of germs or infectious agents—bacteria, viruses, mold—which could produce serious infections if they were to enter the body. Our immune system blocks this invasion. There are also infectious agents called parasites. We do not hear much about parasites anymore, since modern hygienic practices have dramatically reduced their incidence in Western society. There was a time when parasites—worms especially—were common. This was particularly true in warm or temperate climates where people went barefoot, because worms often enter the body from the earth via the skin of the feet.

Over time (millenia) in the course of human evolution, the human body developed a mechanism uniquely suited to combat infestation by worms. This mechanism persists in all of us and involves producing IgE. IgE fastens on white blood cells, called mast cells or basophils; it is present in very small amounts. When the body's immune system sensed an invasion by a parasite, two things happened. First, there was an increase in the production of IgE. Second, there was contact of the invader with the IgE to trigger a release of chemicals that attacked the parasite. This mechanism effectively took care of parasites, but it is flawed in two ways; it is not necessary under contemporary conditions, since worms are pretty much a rarity in North America and the body is tricked into making IgE and discharging chemicals that actually cause allergic symptoms when other foreign substances—pollens, dust, mold, mildew, animal dander, certain foods—enter the body. The major cause of allergic reactions is histamine, one of the chemicals resulting from the IgE and the invader coming together. Histamine triggers the symptoms we see in allergy sufferers—nasal problems, sneezing, wheezing, hives, rashes, and so on.

Therefore, an allergic reaction occurs:

1. When IgE resides on mast cells;
2. When a foreign substance like pollen invades the body;

3. When the immune system (IgE) detects the presence of the invader and releases histamine and other chemicals from certain white (mast) cells;
4. When enough chemicals from inside white cells are released, the allergic symptoms occur locally—on the skin, or in the respiratory, vascular, or digestive system.

People who do not have allergies do not produce enough IgE to trigger the histamine release. This fact puzzles parents who want to know "Why my child?"

Bob Brown is 11 years old, and his brother Joey is 9. They are as alike as two brothers can be. Although Bob is taller, they could readily pass for twins. However, their health histories are very different. Bob suffers from recurrent allergies. It seems sometimes that he is allergic to everything—trees, grasses, pollens, weeds, molds, house dust, and many foods. Joey, on the other hand, is allergic to nothing. They both eat the same things. They grew up in the same house. They attend the same school. They like the same sports and hobbies. Bob owes his allergies to inheriting a special set of genes. These genes were passed from a combination of his mother and his father, and they allow him to produce an excess of IgE. Joey, on the other hand, did not inherit these types of genes and has always been spared from having allergies. The differences between most allergic and nonallergic children rest in their genes.

The fact that allergies are inherited does not mean that if you or your spouse has allergies, your child will necessarily be affected, *nor* does it mean that if you do not have allergies your children will be spared. *Nor* does it mean that if one child has allergies, another child will also turn up with allergies.

What it does mean is that you are more likely to see allergies in your children if one parent has an allergy. If both you and your mate have allergies, it is even more likely that your children will have allergies. There is little you can do to prevent allergies in your child although many studies suggest that breast-feeding may dramatically delay their onset and reduce their severity.

Another aspect of the allergy picture has to do with the differences between children and adults. Vulnerability to allergies is dependent on the age and level of maturation of the individual; children are more susceptible to them. Children are more than just small adults; they are developing and growing. Many of their tissues, organs, and processes are not fully mature. This is important because most materials that cause allergies are either inhaled or eaten. Thus, although children may ingest the same food that adults do, their absorptive and digestive processes are different from those in grown-ups. In children, this immaturity often allows food materials to be absorbed and passed unchanged into the body, whereas in adults, the food materials would be digested more completely. Some foods, especially cow's milk, find it easier to pass undigested into the bodies of children. Similarly, the airways are not fully mature in children, and this condition may permit pollen or other inhaled materials, like dust, to get into the lungs more easily. The entry of these invaders—undigested foods, inhaled materials—sets off the immunologic reaction described earlier, which results in histamine release and the onset of allergic symptoms.

Finally, allergies in children often have widespread ripple effects. Children with recurrent hay fever are more susceptible to earaches, ear infections, and sinus disease; asthmatic children are more often subject to bronchitis and pneumonia; children with eczema are prone to many infections and diseases—even cataracts. Furthermore, any chronically ill child may experience fatigue, tension, depression, restlessness, and sleep disorders.

2

How To Know Whether Your Child Is Allergic

Introduction

Allergies wrongly catch the blame for myriad complaints. Your doctor should be the one to say if your child really has an allergy. However, there are several questions that your doctor should ask to help him/her arrive at a diagnosis—questions you should be prepared to answer.

- What exactly are the sick child's symptoms?
- When, where, and under what circumstances do symptoms show up, and how do they manifest themselves?
- Are the symptoms associated with other factors you can point to like time of the day, weather conditions, season of the year, being outdoors, eating particular foods, wearing apparel, medications, changes in personal habits, or out of the ordinary events?
- Do you, the parents, have a history of allergies? What kind?
- Do any brothers or sisters have allergies? What kind?

Family History of Allergies

The chances that a child will develop an allergy are two to five times greater if either or both of the parents have a history of allergies. For mothers without a history of eczema, the odds are approximately 4 in 100 that their children will show this disease; for mothers who themselves have had eczema, on the average 8 or more in 100 of their children will also experience it. (In both instances, we assume the fathers have no history of eczema.)

11

The chances of an allergic parent having an allergic child are very high; any gambling casino would be ecstatic to operate with odds like that in its favor. However, the appearance of symptoms, whatever they are, in the individual child is unpredictable. If the firstborn is allergic, that does not mean that the second or any other children will necessarily be so troubled.

Heredity is a factor in the transmission of allergic diseases but its effect is variant, and except in the most extraordinary circumstances, should not be an element in deciding whether or not to have children. You should be aware of the existence of this risk factor, however, and be prepared to furnish your obstetrician, or your child's pediatrician, or family physician with information about your allergic history, that of your spouse, your other children, and both sets of grandparents if that information can be obtained.

What Are the Symptoms?

Allergic symptoms most often involve the skin, the upper and lower respiratory systems, and the gastrointestinal tract. Less frequently (and usually as a companion to involvement of these major systems), they may turn up in the eyes or the ears. Rarely, a special and potentially disastrous allergic symptom is a disease called anaphylaxis, or allergic shock, in which the blood pressure falls, the heart rate increases, and the airways constrict.

The most common allergic symptoms that affect these organs or systems are outlined in Table 1; each of the associated allergic diseases named there is discussed in detail in the chapters that make up Part Three of this volume.

Any of these symptoms should alert you to the possibility that an allergy may be responsible; if other, different symptoms show up in the organs or systems listed, something other than an allergy is probably responsible.

The When and How of Allergic Diseases in Children

Whether symptoms originate with an allergy depends to a considerable extent on the age of the child and the way in which symptoms show up and progress. Both of these aspects are dealt with comprehensively in the Chapters comprising Part Three of this volume. Table 2 sketches the typical age of onset, and charts the usual course or progress for the most common allergic diseases in children.

Associated Factors

Allergies grow out of a host of factors or conditions—from the time of the year or today's weather or what your child had for lunch to the arrival of a new pet, the move to a new house or apartment, the use of makeup, even a walk in the park.

Table I
Common Symptoms of Allergic Disease

Organ or system	Type of systems[a]	Possible allergic disease[b]
Skin	Sores	Eczema, contact dermatitis
	Wheals	Hives
	Intense itching	
Upper respiratory tract	Runny nose (clear, thin discharge)	Hay fever (seasonal or chronic)
	Sneezing, itchy throat	
Lower respiratory tract	Cough, thick clingy mucus, wheezing, shortness of breath	Asthma
Gastrointestinal tract	Stomachache	Food allergy
	Constipation	
	Diarrhea	
	Colic	
Ears	Itching or aching	Hay fever
Eyes	Itching, burning, or tearing	Hay fever, allergic conjunctivitis
Mouth and throat	Swelling of mucous tissue	Food allergy, insect stings or bites
Circulatory (vascular) system	Low blood pressure, faintness	Anaphylaxis
		Food allergy

[a]The symptoms listed are possibly the result of allergic disease. However, all of them can be brought on by nonallergic conditions. The mere presence of the symptoms should not be taken as incontrovertible evidence that an allergy is to blame.
[b]Only the most common allergic diseases are represented in the table.

The most common of these allergy associates are named in the Allergy Finder (Fig. 1). If your youngster is troubled with symptoms that might be owing to an allergy, you can use the Finder to narrow down the possible causes and, at the same time, be somewhat more confident about knowing what is causing the symptoms. Carefully maintaining the Allergy Finder and taking it along to your doctor will help in deciding whether or not your child's problems are the result of an allergy.

Directions for Using the Allergy Finder

Fill out the Allergy Finder each day in the evening, just before the child goes to bed. It should take you only a few minutes.

For the Symptoms section, if the child had no symptoms that day, leave the spaces blank; if there were symptoms, indicate what they were (sneezing; runny nose; wheezing; coughing; upset stomach; nausea; diarrhea; and so forth) and then go on to indicate when they appeared, how severe they were, and whether or not they disappeared or persisted and became worse.

Table 2
Allergic Diseases and Their Characteristics

Allergic disease	Usual age of onset	Appearance and progress of symptoms
Eczema	6 months or older	Starts with intense itching accompanied by scratching, restlessness, sleep disturbance; lesions then appear, their character and location dependent on child's age and degree of severity.
Hives	Uncommon before 2 years	Sudden appearance of wheals (slightly raised inflamed areas), followed by intense itching. Wheals usually disappear within a few hours but may migrate to other parts of body.
Seasonal hay fever	4–18 years	Repetitive sneezing with itching of palate, throat, and ear canal; usually seasonal, particularly springtime, and made worse on high-pollen-count and windy days.
Chronic hay fever	4–18 years	Repetitive year-round sneezing, often worse indoors and when exposed to dust. Sneezing with throat, palate, and ear canal itching; often associated with clogged ears and sinusitis.
Asthma	18 months to any age	Shortness of breath, coughing, wheezing.
Food allergy	Birth to any age	Diarrhea, colic; can involve almost any organ or system in the body, triggering hay fever, hives, eczema, or asthma.

14

For all other sections, check every item for which you have a "yes" answer that day. In the Foods section make a special effort to record everything that the child consumed.

To interpret the form, at the end of the week, count the number of check marks that you have made for each entry and record the number in the Total column at the right.

Then relate the entries in the Symptoms section to those in all of the other sections: For example, if you checked no symptoms all week, what other categories or items had no check that week? If the child did have symptoms, which of the other boxes were also checked on the day before or on the day the symptoms showed? If the child was troubled with symptoms throughout the whole week, which boxes had checks every day? Write any suspected match-up of symptoms and causes below:

Dates	Symptoms?	Possible Causes
_____	_____	_____
_____	_____	_____
_____	_____	_____
_____	_____	_____
_____	_____	_____

It may be necessary to keep the Allergy Finder for a number of weeks, so we encourage you to photocopy the Finder beforehand. Bring the completed form to your doctor; it will help him or her figure out what is wrong with your child.

The Doctor's Role

For confident diagnosis of allergy in your child and prescription of appropriate remedies, you need to see your doctor. Chapter 22 tells you how to go about choosing a physician and describes the procedures he or she will follow in treating your youngster. In summary, your doctor should:

1. Take a good, detailed history.
2. Make a complete, thorough physical examination that includes measures of height, weight, blood pressure, inspection of ears, nose, eyes, mouth, throat, listening to heart and lungs, and close examination of skin plus collecting information on general health practices, diet, sleep, exercise, and so on.(These first two steps, carefully done, are often enough to provide a firm diagnosis. If they do not, then some of the following tests may be required.)
3. Skin (called scratch, prick, or intradermal) tests done in the doctor's office to detect sensitivity to substances possibly causing the allergic reaction. (Skin testing should be used with caution; it

is not appropriate for young children, if eczema is present, or for any child who is having an allergic flare-up or asthma attack at the time of testing.)

4. Laboratory blood tests (called RAST or FAST) that determine the presence of heightened levels of IgE. These tests can confirm that an IgE or allergic antibody is present, but do not pin down the cause any better than skin tests.

5. Challenge tests, usually done in the hospital or clinic. These tests directly assess the reaction to suspected allergens. They entail some risks and are not appropriate for all allergic reactions.

Allergies and Allergy Imposters

Allergies unfairly catch the blame for too many complaints. "I think he is allergic to something," a parent may say to explain a child's skin irritation, chronic runny nose, intestinal upset, headache, or virtually any other ailment to which the body is subject.

There are a number of good reasons for this unfortunate tendency toward indiscriminate labeling. "Allergy" has gradually taken on a meaning much broader than its original one. You have doubtless heard, seen, or perhaps even light-heartedly made statements like these: "I'm allergic to my boss," "my teacher," "my in-laws," "math," "Christmas." In this context you declare yourself "allergic" to any source of discomfort, annoyance, or frustration, and you may also diagnose "allergy" when troubled with any symptom or condition whose cause is unknown to you.

> Lucy chain smokes. Whenever she lights up, her 6-year-old son Eric begins coughing. She is convinced that Eric is allergic to smoke. Totally addicted, she cannot give up cigarettes, and Eric cannot seem to stop coughing. In desperation she turns to an allergist hoping that Eric will be able to get allergy shots to relieve his condition. The allergist patiently tries to explain that Eric is not allergic to the smoke. It is merely an irritant that is noxious for his lungs. Lucy cannot seem to understand. "I know he is allergic to smoke," she says. "I know, because he coughs when I smoke."

Doctors have also contributed to the terminological muddle. They have used the word loosely, sometimes calling a reaction allergic when it is really the result of something else which they consider too difficult or involved to explain to the patient. What they often mean is that you have an intolerance.

> Bob loves to eat at Taco Bell, and he likes to eat what his friends do. Within an hour after eating tacos with jalapenos, Bob will turn up with a major stomachache. His mother thinks he is allergic to something in Taco Bell. However, Bob is not allergic to either franchise Mexican restaurants or spicy food; rather his body has an intolerance to the spices.

Then there is the scenario that goes like this: Your child has a recurring problem—for instance, diarrhea, or constipation, a skin rash, a chronic runny nose, ear infections. You take the child to the doctor, who runs a diagnostic test. The test is inconclusive. "Probably an allergy" the doctor says and sends you to a specialist who orders more tests, finds nothing clear-cut, but still declares that the symptoms are owing to an allergic reaction for which treatment is prescribed and which may or may not work. In instances like these, allergy comes to be either a diagnostic wastebasket into which unexplained symptoms are dumped or it refers to symptoms that look as if they ought to be allergic, but are really attributable to an allergy imposter.

> Dr. Paul is a wonderful old-fashioned general practitioner. Over the years he has learned that he does not have everything to offer all patients, but he has always felt obliged to tell his patients what the trouble is—to give them a diagnosis. One of his patients is Jackie Fitzgerald, a teenager. Jackie is chronically constipated and very troubled and embarrassed by her stubborn condition. Dr. Paul checked her carefully, recommended that she take a glass of prune juice each morning, and added by way of explanation and reassurance, "Jackie, you're probably just allergic to certain foods." Unfortunately, although the prune juice treatment worked just fine, Jackie became obsessed with the gratuitous suggestion that her problem was rooted in an allergy. She went on a protracted, exhaustive food elimination diet that proved totally uninformative; she and her parents spent serious money on a useless collection of books on food allergies and allergy-free diets; and she developed a phobia about foods that persists to this day. The doctor's careless, unreflective attribution of the problem to "allergy" played havoc with Jackie.

Allergic reactions are expressed in a limited number of symptoms— the most common ones are named and discussed in Part Three of this volume. Most of these symptoms can also be allergy imposters, that is, they can be the outcome of nonallergic reactions. For example, suppose your 2 year-old is subject to frequent ear infections. The principal reason for ear infections in young children is blockage, inflammation, and infection in the eustachian tube. The eustachian tube is a pipe that links the nose to the eardrum; if the tube becomes inflamed, as is often the case during a cold, normal drainage is hindered. Fluid builds up, bacteria invade and multiply, and an ear infection develops. In this instance, the symptoms are allergy imposters.

Exactly the same symptoms can be caused by a eustachian tube closed by hay fever, an allergic condition that can and often does trigger a chain of events identical to those associated with a cold.

It may not seem all that important to make the distinction between earaches caused by allergy and those caused by an allergy imposter. The pain, the crying, the distress, and the treatment for the condition are the same regardless of cause. However, knowing the underlying reason is crucial, because with that knowledge, the parent is helped to forestall possible future episodes and to deal with them efficiently and intelligently if they do recur.

Allergy, Allergy Imposters, and Physical Maturation

As it happens, the physical changes that children experience as they pass through the stages from newborn baby to adolescent are implicated in the allergy-imposter confusion.

- Earaches become less frequent and severe as the child matures and the eustachian tube enlarges.
- Colic or gastric upsets gradually disappear as the digestive system matures to the point where it can handle milk efficiently.
- Episodes of wheezing and asthma tend to become less severe or vanish altogether as the airways in the respiratory system enlarge.

Thus, many childhood symptoms—whether allergy-caused or simply allergy-like—moderate or disappear as the physical development of the child proceeds or as the immunological system matures. (Infants are apt to have 10 or more colds a year; the figure drops to 4 or 5 in primary school youngsters. Exposure and repeated infection help build resistance.)

For _____ (Name) Week of _____ (Month) to _____ (Dates) 19___

	Mon	Tue	Wed	Thu	Fri	Sat	Sun	Total
WHAT WERE THE SYMPTOMS?								
WHEN DID THE SYMPTOMS SHOW?								
Morning								
Afternoon								
Evening								
During the night								
HOW SEVERE WERE THE SYMPTOMS?								
No symptoms seen								
Mild								
Moderate								
Severe								
DID THE SYMPTOMS								
Disappear?								
Disappear and return?								
Persist?								
Persist and worsen?								
WAS THE WEATHER								
Cold?								
Snowy/Rainy?								
Windy?								
Hot/Humid?								

Fig. 1. Part 1

19

	Mon	Tue	Wed	Thu	Fri	Sat	Sun	Total
DID THE CHILD HAVE ANY INFECTIONS?								
Cold								
Flu								
Sinusitis								
Other*								
WHERE DID THE CHILD GO? WHAT DID HE OR SHE DO?								
Daycare								
Preschool								
School								
Home								
Work								
Travel/Dine Out/Recreation								
Played outside								
Exercised vigorously								
Other*								
WAS THE CHILD EXPOSED TO								
Smoke/tobacco?								
Dust/Pollen?								
Mold/Dampness								
Auto emissions?								
Other fumes?								
Animals/Pets?								
Chemicals or solvents?								
Other airborne irritants?*								
DID THE CHILD USE, WEAR, OR COME IN CONTACT WITH								
Cigarettes?								
Detergents/Soaps?								
Perfume/Cosmetics?								
Bath preparations?								
Wool/fur/leather?								
Jewelry?								
Poison oak, ivy, sumac?								
Insecticides or other chemicals?								
Other suspected triggers?*								

*Specify.

Fig. 1. (continued) Part 2

20

	Mon	Tue	Wed	Thu	Fri	Sat	Sun	Total
DID THE CHILD TAKE ANY DRUGS OR MEDICATIONS?								
Aspirin								
Other pain or headache remedy*								
Cold medicine*								
Nose drops*								
Skin medication*								
Antibiotics*								
Other*								
DID THE CHILD EXPERIENCE ANY UNUSUAL STRESS, TENSION, ANXIETY, OR CONFLICT?								
WHAT DID THE CHILD EAT?								
Grains or cereals (breads, pastries, breakfast foods)								
Milk or milk products (ice cream, cheese, sour cream, cottage cheese, yogurt, etc.)								
Eggs/egg products								
Poultry								
Meats (fresh or processed)								
Fish or shellfish								
Raw fruits or vegetables								
Snacks, including candies								
Chocolate								
Nuts or nut butter								
Popcorn								
Chewing gum								
Beverages, including tea								
coffee								
cola/soda								
beer, wine, or other alcohol								

*Specify.

Fig. 1. (continued) Part 3

21

3

Guiding Your Allergic Child into the Mainstream

We designed this book to help parents recognize, manage, and prevent their children's allergic problems. Much of what we discuss concerns avoiding allergen contact or exposure at home. However, as every parent realizes, a child's universe begins expanding from the day of birth, continually widening with exposure to different environments, new situations, and changed responsibilities. During their formative years, children spend many hours in school or at the homes of friends; those with working parents have lengthy periods of time at home, alone; they may celebrate holidays or special occasions more actively than adults do; they attend summer camp, travel, or vacation with their families. For the allergic child, each of these aspects of growing up represents a special circumstance and poses certain risks—risks that can be met and countered with careful planning and forethought.

General Health Problems

Although there are any number of problems that can grow out of allergic conditions, the most common and troublesome ones are associated with the child's general health or school performance. It is important to recognize and manage general health problems arising out of allergic conditions that occur often enough to be a matter of concern to parents. These can range from chronic eye or ear problems to low energy level or little resistance to recurring infections, like colds or flu, or to chronic ones, like sinusitis. Here are some of the things parents can do to deal effectively with the possibility that an allergy has in some way undermined the child's general health:

1. Monitor the child's behavior to the extent that you can become aware of any substantial departures from the ordinary—lassitude,

apathy, hyperactivity, change in sleep patterns or needs, complaints about not feeling well, stomachache, headache, and so forth. (Try to keep your eye on the child without becoming obsessive or overly solicitous about it; these are mistakes that carry their own separate recipes for disaster.)

2. If the atypical behavior persists for more than a day or two, talk openly and matter-of-factly with the youngster about it. If necessary, check the child's temperature, breathing, and so on.

3. Be alert to the fact that some allergy medications can produce the symptoms named above. Review the child's medication regime and find out their possible side effects. In general, do not administer medications unless they are professionally prescribed and avoid the pitfalls of buying ineffective over-the-counter medications.

Ginny, a consistent honor roll student, has had hay fever for years. This past spring, however, she had difficulty concentrating and her grades dropped markedly. Her mother sent her for an evaluation, convinced the allergy caused her slump. Ginny's problem was not her allergies; instead the culprit was the over-the-counter antihistamine (chlortrimetron) she was taking. Ginny's new HMO only provided cost-cutting older medicines, not the newer, better, more expensive ones that do not carry the negative side effects like those Ginny suffered.

4. Confer with your doctor, describing the symptoms fully (onset, nature, severity, what you have done about them), and request and act on the doctor's recommendations.

School Problems

Depending on the allergy or allergies, life at school can present serious complications to families with allergic children. The nature of your child's allergies—asthma, eczema, hay fever, and so forth—will have you thinking about whether or not to use the cafeteria, wondering about physical education, field trips, school or class parties, the advisability of taking certain subjects, the extent of contact with other children, and so on. To deal with these issues effectively, it is extremely important that you and your child know as much as possible about the causes and methods of controlling allergies. Here are some questions you should consider, have the answers to, and discuss with school authorities (principal, teachers, counselor, nurse) before school even starts.

1. Do your child's allergies, especially asthma, appear during or get worse with exercise?

2. Do sharp or pungent odors trigger or intensify your child's symptoms?

3. Does soap cause skin irritation or eczema in your child?

4. Does your child react negatively to some foods?
5. Does exposure to heat or dust make your child's symptoms get worse?
6. Does handling clay, glue, or other substances cause contact allergies (dermatitis) in your child?
7. Does your child feel troubled or conspicuous at being left out of certain programs or activities?
8. Do you, the child, and school officials know what to do about the foregoing problems?
9. Do you know the school policy about administering medication during the school day? Have you worked out a mutually satisfactory and thoroughly understood procedure for getting medication to the child when it is needed?
10. Do you, the school, and the child know what to do if the child develops symptoms at school? Have you agreed on a procedure to follow if symptoms intensify or become serious? What is their policy for managing medical emergencies?

Overall School Performance

Allergies, especially hay fever and asthma, can pull down school performance either directly by forcing frequent, extended absences, or indirectly by requiring medication that makes the child hyperactive or drowsy and inattentive. Get to know your child's abilities and level of performance through your own observations, consultation with teachers and counselor, and familiarity with past academic record. If grades start sliding, find out why by talking with the child and the teacher or teachers involved. Learn exactly what is happening and why. Asking the child (and teachers) to describe specific events, or behavior will probably lead to some hunches about the reasons for the fall-off. Strive to establish the nature of the difficulty and, in cooperation with child and teacher, work toward a solution that everyone can live with.

Help the child by identifying the reason for the poor performance—if that is truly what it is—and getting rid of it. Scrupulously avoid doing the work for the child. That will do nothing at all to solve whatever academic difficulties he or she is having and it sets a bad precedent for later difficulties, should they occur.

Physical Education

Physical education is an important part of the school curriculum. Although there are some children who have physical disabilities that make it impossible for them to participate in such programs, this is not the case for children with allergies. Youngsters with hay fever, eczema, or even those with asthma may participate in physical education provided common sense precautions and limitations are observed. First, if your child has eczema and washes or showers after exercise, it is important to avoid all soaps without fail or use nonsoap skin cleansers. Children are often very self-conscious about not using soap in a communal situation, and to avoid teasing and embarrassment, they may soap up like the rest of the kids. The child should be helped by you and the teacher to withstand this sort of pressure.

> Andy has had eczema for as long as he can remember. Andy resents his mother's continual harping about avoiding soap. He is now 13 and on the school basketball team. His eczema has been pretty well controlled for years. However, in the shower after practice, he did like the rest of the guys, lathering himself with soap. Three days later, his skin was painfully red and dry. A day after that the skin started to crack and small localized infections sprouted. Finally Andy could stand it no longer and showed the sores to his mother. She packed him off to their dermatologist who prescribed an aggressive treatment of steroid creams and lectured Andy sharply.

Children with hay fever can exercise and play with the same intensity as any other children. Those receiving good medical treatment for their hay fever should have no problems whatsoever, but if your child is in the throes of a hay fever attack, it is best that he or she stay quiet and indoors, off the playground, or out of the gym until medication brings the symptoms under firm control.

As we noted above with Ginny, some antihistamines, particularly older ones, prescribed for mild cases of hay fever may make children sleepy, adversely affect school performance, and interfere with attentiveness at school. The school should know if your child is on antihistamines; we discuss this issue at length in Chapter 12. We do not recommend drugs that sedate children!

Children with asthma are in by far the worst situation when it comes to manifesting symptoms at school. Even mild exercise may trigger some degree of wheezing in virtually every asthmatic child. This should be forestalled; often judicious use of medication before exercise will suppress symptoms. If your child starts to wheeze or wheezes more severely during exercise, it is prudent to avoid hard physical exertion. Redirection into exercises or activities that are more appropriate for asthmatic children would be helpful; swimming is, by far, the most suitable activity for asthmatic children, but most middle and high schools of any size will be able to offer "adaptive" physical education activities for children unable to do the regular program comfortably. Your child should get advice from the doctor about steps to take to prevent exercise-induced asthma.

Other Classes

We believe that children with allergies should be given the opportunity to take the full spectrum of courses and that their academic choices not be limited because of their illness. Fortunately, for the vast majority of allergic children this is not an issue, because appropriate and timely use of medication can effectively prevent symptoms from developing.

However, strong, pungent fumes or odors can trigger asthma or other allergies. Most commonly, this occurs in the high school or college chemistry lab where the fumes emitted can be strong enough to bring on wheezing. The villains here are mainly sulfur dioxide or hydrogen sulfide, which smells like rotten eggs. To prevent reactions, wearing a paper mask is sometimes all it takes; in other instances, a more aggressive medication program may be necessary. All asthmatic children should be wary of chemistry laboratories.

> Anne did so well in math and science that she was accepted for a special National Science Foundation program for bright high school kids at the University of California at Berkeley. During her first week of classes, she was assigned to work in an organic chemistry lab. Although most of the chemical exercises took place under special hoods where the gases are sucked away and dispersed outside, the lab still smelled of acids and ethers, esters, and sulfur. Anne, who had suffered from asthma during childhood, suddenly found herself coughing during each chemistry lab. Although it was only a cough, she was uncomfortable and did feel her chest getting tight. She did not think it was asthma because she remembered hearing herself wheeze as a child and there were no wheezes this time. Nonetheless, she went to the Student Health Center where the doctor listened to her with a stethoscope. His first question was: "Have you ever been told you have asthma?" Anne could not believe her ears. She had not had a wheeze in over 6 years. They discussed the situation and the fact that the cough seemed to get worse in the chemistry lab. The doctor suggested a special mask. Anne used it and had no problems thereafter.

Physical contact with a wide range of substances at school can also trigger allergic symptoms. In younger children, paints, pastes, glues, or modeling clay can and often do bring on contact dermatitis. In older children, classes in art, shop, and cooking expose them to unusual dusts (wood; flour) and fumes (solder flux, glue, paint). Cleaning solutions, and a variety of other materials can bring on dermatitis, as well as nasal or respiratory problems. Excessive heat can intensify eczema; dust from sweeping, chalkboard, playground, or heating vents can provoke hay fever or asthma; air-conditioning units can spew asthma or hay fever-causing mold into the environment. Anything at all that causes allergies at home—plus the great opportunity the school affords for the transmission of colds and respiratory infections—can turn up at school.

The possible causes of allergies and methods of avoiding them are covered in Part Two of this volume. Your job, as parent, is to be alert to the appearance of symptoms and to review your child's activities carefully. (*This may well be the hardest part of your job!* Most children are infuriatingly laconic when asked to talk about their activities in school. Pin down the cause of the reaction, then take action to treat the symptoms, and in cooperation with the school, remove or avoid their cause or causes.)

Other Risks at School

For children with serious food hypersensitivities, the school lunch represents a problem. Sometimes it is hard to know what is in school cafeteria food. If your child reacts to some common foods like flour, peanut butter, milk, and so forth, it may be appropriate to pack a lunch and send it along to school with the youngster, or to teach the child to do that himself or herself.

Perhaps a more important problem for children in school, though, is the intense peer pressure not to be different. This is reflected in the extraordinary and sometimes dangerous lengths kids will go to in order to seem just like everybody else. In teenaged girls, for instance, there has recently been an enormous increase in the use of beauty aids—face and eye makeup, shampoos, scents, fingernail preparations. In girls with eczema or contact dermatitis the push to look made-up like everyone else can provoke or aggravate skin problems tragically.

For both boys and girls, there is pressure to drink alcohol, to smoke, sniff, or snort substances, and to wear certain kinds of clothes. The first two activities are illegal as well as dangerous for any child; for allergic children they can be exceptionally hazardous—in some instances lethal. Also, in certain allergic youngsters, even wearing the "right" kinds of clothes—rubber, wool, plastics, leather—can bring on troublesome skin reactions.

Here you, the parents, have to remind the child of his or her uniqueness and vulnerability, and the need to take appropriate precautions. Worse, you have to do it without pushing the child into rebellion, withdrawal, or overdependence on you.

At Homes of Friends

When visiting or sleeping over at a friend's house, the allergic child and the parents of the friend need to know how to deal with any potential problems that may erupt. You should see to it that your child carries along whatever is needed to avoid or manage difficulties encountered at the friend's house, including medications and any other special preparations or equipment required for allergy treatment. Be very careful about dogs and cats. For children with allergies, pets are not their best friend. The other parents should be aware (beforehand) of the allergy, how it manifests itself, what triggers it—foods, exercise, pets, whatever—and what to do if anything happens. Your child can help by knowing how too and behaving responsibly in this unfamiliar environment. Be very vocal if your child has a food allergy.

Billy has severe allergies to peanuts. He went to a birthday party and ate a piece of the birthday cake. Almost immediately he began wheezing and could not catch his breath. 911 was called, and he was rushed to the ER where fortunately he received successful treatment. On analysis, there were no nuts in the birthday cake, but the knife that cut the cake had been used earlier to make a peanut butter sandwich, and the leavings came off on Billy's piece.

At Home Alone

Millions of children are "latchkey kids," returning to an empty home while parent or parents are away at work. In addition to the routine precautions and communication strategies that this situation demands, allergic latchkey kids have to be responsible for watching out for their allergies. They should know what they must do to avoid or control triggers, when, how, and how much to medicate, and what activities are permissible. Allergic children live in a world with limits. Your job is to teach them these boundaries. Small contributions on your part can help greatly; for example, if your child has food allergies, preparing the ritual after-school snack beforehand and leaving it in a special place in the refrigerator will guard against eating something that may bring on wheezing, hives, stomach upset, or any of the other symptoms that food allergy produces.

Where substantial risk to the child is involved—shock reactions to foods, insect stings, severe wheezing brought on by exertion or infection, and so on—you need to take two additional precautions. First, recruit someone dependable like a neighbor or nearby relative who is willing and trained (by you) to know exactly what to do and can minister to the child in an emergency. Instruct the child to call this emergency care provider if anything goes wrong. Second, arrange it so that people know where and how you can be reached at work if that should become necessary. Have a written procedures list to follow for allergic emergencies.

Holidays

Holidays are risky times for any child who, in addition to overdosing on food, activity, and excitement, is likely to encounter different foods in unfamiliar settings; for allergic youngsters, the risks are even higher.

Randy, an 8-year-old, has had asthma since he was 2. His mother has noticed that he always gets worse right around Christmas. The doctor suggested that he might be allergic to the Christmas tree. In fact, one year they had an outdoor Christmas tree and Randy was better during that season, although he continued to wheeze somewhat. The doctor also asked about unusual activities restricted to the season. "We keep a fire going in the fireplace and we use a lot of candles, scented ones," Randy's Mom said. "Cut them out next time and see what happens" the doctor advised. It was not like their traditional Christmas: No tree, no cheerful fire crackling in the fireplace, no candles. No asthma either.

In most instances, if you know what triggers your child's allergies, and what you and your child must do to avoid and treat them, you can get through any holiday by being watchful and imposing and enforcing whatever allergy-dodging steps are necessary. This may put a mild damper on the festivities, but a safe and sane celebration is clearly to be preferred to one where flaring allergies ruin everyone's fun.

Traveling

Travel, particularly the kind that involves staying in strange places, eating out-of-the-ordinary foods, or engaging in unaccustomed activities, can be accompanied by the development of symptoms. If you have an allergic child, *never* leave home on a trip without carrying an adequate supply of medicine. Also, never entrust your medicines to a checked suitcase. Carry them with you.

As far as accommodations are concerned, depending on the allergy and its trigger, you may want to look for places to stay that do not admit pets, that offer tobacco-free rooms, or that on inspection (you can and should ask to look at the room before renting it) seem to be clean and mold-free. If the problem is not the kind that can be spotted by mere inspection, ask the innkeeper the relevant questions.

> Lew, 10, has an acute hypersensitivity reaction to fabric softeners, the strips of chemically treated perfumed paper thrown into a clothes dryer to make the wash soft and "fragrant." Whenever he touches anything that has been in contact with one of these chemicals—sheets, pillow cases, towels, clothing—he breaks out with a severe case of hives. From bitter experience, Lew's parents have learned to ask first if the motel uses fabric softeners on the sheets and towels. If the answer is "Yes" or "I do not know," they find another place.

Strange foods (or additives) can also cause problems to the unwary. This possible source of difficulty can be avoided to an extent by doing what you can (and what you can do is considerable) to supply your own food as you go. However, if your family's mode of travel entails driving day and night, straight through, stopping only to refuel or to get food at a fast-food place, expect problems.

What is true of public accommodations is also true of public transportation. Buses, planes, and trains are generally inadequately ventilated and may be contaminated with pollutants. Virtually every public seat in an airport or train station is filled with animal dander. The dander is carried on the clothes of fellow passengers.

Note, also, that federal and state regulations prohibit smoking on domestic airline flights. Some international flights still permit smoking, but a few carriers have outlawed it altogether. If necessary, seek out and patronize health-conscious firms. Furthermore, if a complaint becomes necessary, take it to the highest level, the president or chief executive officer of the company. It will not help your child this trip but long-run policy changes may result. If you get sick on an airline and do not get a satisfactory response, think about seeing your attorney. That may be the only way to get the attention your child's (and other children's) health deserves.

The food on board or in the terminals or depots is likely to have been prepared well in advance, and laced with salt and preservatives. It is possible to order special vegetarian or kosher meals beforehand if traveling by air, but there are no special provisions for the allergic traveler whose only recourse is to beware. Airlines are totally unprepared for allergic reactions on board. As already emphasized, carry your medicines with you. Do not check them!

Summer Camp

Summer camp is a memorable experience in any case; it is particularly worthwhile for children with allergies, especially asthma. Many years ago, a Denver-based group began a summer camp called Camp Broncho, to "buck" bronchial asthma; they called the campers "bucking bronchos." This was a daring and innovative move at the time; since then, respiratory societies and lung associations all over America have promoted the use of summer camps for children with asthma, and they will know of local summer camps geared to the needs of asthmatic kids. They are usually attended by physicians who volunteer their time, and nursing supervision is provided so that the children are monitored and keep up with their medicine. The camps are extraordinarily helpful for several reasons:

1. Camps give parents time away from their chronically asthmatic children.
2. Asthmatic children meet and learn from one another.
3. Children develop self-esteem and a sense of competency, control over their disease, and self-worth.
4. Camps provide sound, protective, fun-filled environments.
5. Camps teach children to swim. Swimming is the only form of exercise that does not make asthma worse.

Your local lung association will be able to direct you to summer camps for asthmatic youngsters.

Special Problems of Allergic Children

Allergic kids are like other children and need to and can be treated like other youngsters without making any great to-do or fuss about their condition.

They experience all of the events of growing up in common with other children, and for the most part, need neither shielding from nor special help with this stream of developments. There are a few things that sometimes roughen the path a bit, and these possible complications are covered in this section.

In later chapters we deal with the special significance headaches (Chapter 18), fever (Chapter 19), and colds (Chapter 20) hold for allergic youngsters. Apart from these complaints, children in general are also quite prone to injuries, fungus infections, skin eruptions, dental problems, and there is also the real possibility of experimentation with drugs or alcohol.

Injuries (cuts and lacerations, sprains, fractures) are a routine feature of growing up. They themselves do not represent an added hazard to allergic children, but their treatment can sometimes precipitate problems. Depending on the severity of the injury, it may be necessary to prescribe pain relievers, antibiotics (to guard against infection), or to give a tetanus booster.

Antipain medication, anything that contains aspirin or codeine, should be administered cautiously to allergic kids, and should absolutely not be given to asthmatics where the drug can either trigger the reaction (aspirin) or depress the respiratory system (codeine). Tetanus shots do not in themselves carry any threat to allergic children but if the child dreads the needle, the fear can sometimes affect breathing and intensify respiratory problems.

Antibiotics, especially penicillin, are notorious triggers of allergic reactions, and should be administered only if the need for them is clear and then only if the physician knows that your child has allergies.

Fungus infections, especially of feet and hands, are a routine nuisance in children. For the most part, they can be managed readily by careful washing, and by keeping the affected areas dry and open to the air as much as possible. Fungus infections (and some of the many over-the-counter medications available for the treatment of athletes' food, jock itch, and other variations on fungus infections) sometimes interact with existing skin allergies, notably eczema and allergic contact dermatitis, and need to be treated carefully and as conservatively as possible.

Skin eruptions, pimples and acne, are a matter of great concern to many adolescents. For the most part, these blemishes are self-limiting, clearing up on their own in time. There is a huge arsenal of topical medications around to treat these conditions, some of them fairly effective, but most of them without merit. However, the treatments (and the alternative tactic of covering the sores with makeup) can cause hypersensitivity or allergic reactions (triggering allergic contact dermatitis; worsening eczema) and probably ought to be avoided by teenagers with allergy-related skin problems.

Dental problems are the bane of everyone's existence. Allergic kids are going to need to have their teeth cleaned, cavities filled, and in some instances, extractions made and orthodontic work carried out. Where dental work is concerned, there are a few things that parents of allergic kids should be alert to. The anesthetics used to block pain (novocaine or other "caines") can trigger hives or more serious shock reactions in some susceptible individuals; postoperative pain remedies (as with injuries) can also represent a possible source of difficulty.

Drugs and alcohol are bad news for anyone, but they carry added dangers for allergic kids. Alcohol and some recreational drugs can greatly compromise the respiratory and vascular systems, and represent a real danger to asthmatics especially.

Other Problems

In addition to the special problems and risks that ordinary diseases or conditions may represent to allergic kids, there is the hard fact that they may have to be denied certain kinds of experiences that other children are free to enjoy. Prominent among these deprivations is the freedom to have and enjoy pets. For children who react to respiratory allergens, the plea to keep a dog or cat or horse or bird should be denied, kindly but firmly and with a sympathetic explanation. Where a pet is already on the scene and causing problems, find it a good foster home; this can be a hard, bitter step to take, especially where the child is attached to the animal, but keeping it would only bring you and the child a different kind of grief.

It may also be necessary to exercise a lot of care about the kinds of toys an allergic youngster has; for kids with respiratory allergies, soft, cuddly dolls—dust-catching teddy bears, giant pandas, and other plush playmates especially—may have to be returned to the wild. This may cause a crisis, but it, too, will pass.

It can help to avoid misunderstanding and disappointment if gift-givers (grandparents, especially) are told about the toys and gifts that would be inappropriate—and appropriate—for the allergic child.

Teaching Allergic Offspring How to Act Judiciously and Competently on Their Own

It has been found that even very young children—4- and 5-year-olds—can, with proper coaching, learn to manage their own allergies competently. This is especially true for asthmatic children—so true, in fact, that there are a number of brief self-management programs that have been developed especially to help asthmatic children deal with their symptoms. Your local Lung Association or HMO will know of these offerings.

Children who have other kinds of allergies than asthma do not have the advantage of being able to participate in such ready-made programs. Notwithstanding, parents can do an effective job of teaching their children how to manage their allergic symptoms. In doing this, there are several important precepts you must keep in mind.

1. The child has to know exactly what the allergy is, what triggers it, and what to do to avoid its cause or causes.
2. The parents and other health care providers have to be willing and able to take the time and expend the energy to learn and then transmit avoidance and treatment strategies in terms that the child fully understands and can follow. It is useful, after providing the information, to set a situation in which the child might realistically find himself or herself (or has already been in) and ask, "What are the things you should do?" Repetition and positive reinforcement ("That's fine!" "Exactly right!") are important in ensuring the success of this phase of the learning program.
3. Parents and health care providers must show the child how to go about making his or her own independent health care decisions, give the child the freedom and the opportunity to make such decisions, and review the decisions and their outcomes carefully. This is probably the most difficult step of all for parents who, not wanting to put the child at risk, are inclined to make these sorts of decisions themselves without consulting the child, or worse, strive to create an environment altogether free of hazards. This excess solitude and lack of confidence in the capacity of the child to act intelligently in his or her own behalf tends to foster long-term and sometimes crippling dependence on the parents and certainly interferes with the child's need to be self-reliant.

Most childhood allergies ease up or disappear during the process of growing up. Where the allergic condition is chronic and persistent, medications and other preventive or avoidance tactics can usually hold the symptoms in check. In short, where parent and child are informed, alert, and thoughtful, allergic children, even those moderately to severely troubled, can and should be helped and encouraged to do the sorts of things nonallergic youngsters do. The suggestions we have outlined here are designed to help parents help their allergic kids to venture into the mainstream of youthful life safely and enjoyably.

Illicit Drugs

Whether taken by nose, mouth, or injection, illicit drugs damage the body. Of all these destroyers, alcohol probably delivers the most aggregate damage and is most often abused by children but other substances—marijuana, amphetamines, cocaine in its various forms, heroin, glues, and myriad other mind benders—are out there for the taking. They are bad for anyone; for allergic kids, they can add up to serious or even lethal bad news, triggering (depending on method of use) catastrophic respiratory or vascular collapse, ugly skin conditions, and severe and chronic damage to bodily systems or organs.

> Bert, a college sophomore, takes his recurring nose bleeds to the Health Service. The doctor there takes a look, and asks, "Do you do coke?" He knew very well that Bert was a user because the drug had burned a hole in Bert's septum. At first Bert weakly denied he was a coke head, but he realized right then he was found out and that he had a serious problem. The Health Center was able to get Bert into a detox and treatment program that seems to have helped him clean up his act.

In addition to the drugs alone, some, like alcohol or marijuana, carry additives or contaminants that spell trouble for the allergic youngster. Sulfites added to wines or beer ratchet up asthma, as do the herbicides and pesticides that accompany marijuana. Dope producers or dealers are not into "natural" or "organic."

Children need to know and be warned of the dangers of drugs. They need to be watched for signs of drug use, and they need to be talked to openly of the Pandora's box that drug use can open—all the way from dependence, to lifelong suffering with hepatitis C to HIV and AIDS from a contaminated needle. It is the parents' responsibility to know and to warn their children of these dangers.

Part Two

What Are Allergies' Triggers and How Can I Avoid or Control Them Effectively?

4

Food and Food Additives

Almost everyone has at one time or another had a reaction that they chose to call a food allergy. This near-universal claim needs to be scrutinized more closely. Take the word "food." Food is actually not only the name of whatever is eaten but all of the materials used to prepare, preserve, and color it, plus residue from packaging or storage materials, and contaminants like pesticides, herbicides, and insect or rodent leavings and remains.

Identifying and then dealing with food allergies or intolerances are one of the more complex and difficult areas in the whole field of allergy. This chapter simply identifies some of the more common causes of these food-linked symptoms, tells how they are expressed, and discusses the symptoms, diagnosis, and treatment of these conditions.

A food allergy is an immune-mediated reaction by the body against the foodstuff itself or something else contained in it. (*See* Chapter 1 for more on the nature of an allergy.)

Actually, what is popularly called a food allergy is, in almost all cases, an "intolerance," a local irritant effect like the heartburn from spicy foods, a headache from too much wine, or diarrhea from too many prunes. Perhaps 1% of all reactions to foods are true allergies; the rest are intolerances, something consumed that did not agree with us or carried distressing side effects.

The bulk of true allergic reactions to food are found in children. As with other allergies, there is an anatomical reason for this. Food is taken into the mouth either in liquid or semiliquid form, or is so rendered by the process of chewing. It then passes along to the stomach and intestine where digestion takes place and the material is broken down into subunits or very "short" chemicals.

These chemicals are then absorbed into the body where they fuel our cells. In infants and toddlers, the intestines are immature, not yet completely developed, and they permit the absorption of "larger" chemicals or actual bits of the food itself. These "larger" chemicals from food are seen by the body's immune system as invaders, and the immune response is triggered.

Milk offers a good example of how all this happens. When adults drink milk, its principal proteins are rapidly broken down by the stomach, leaving only the "short" chemicals; in children minute quantities of the whole, undigested proteins can sometimes be detected in the blood.

Symptoms of Food Allergy or Intolerance

Food (or whatever else food contains) can affect almost any organ or system of the body, and the symptoms can take an astonishing variety of forms, some of them bearing what seems like little or no rational connection to their actual cause.

Apart from the gastrointestinal symptoms that are the most frequent result of food intolerance in young children, they can also be expressed directly (triggering hives and rashes) or indirectly (making eczema worse) as skin disorders; respiratory problems, especially wheezing and shortness of breath; vascular complications ranging from mild headache to sudden, catastrophic drop in blood pressure; itching and swelling of mucous tissue, especially of the throat (palate) or lips; and abdominal pain.

The onset can be sudden or gradual and not necessarily limited to one organ or area; hives and wheezing and/or vascular problems often occur together.

The duration of symptoms can be short-lived, lasting only for a brief period of time, vanishing in a period of an hour or two, or they can persist for days and be responsible for a period of prolonged and acute distress. Adverse reactions to food, in short, add up to a complicated many-stranded puzzle.

Diagnostic Procedures for Establishing the Cause of Food Allergies or Intolerances

Because of the variety of symptoms food intolerances can take and then unpredictable onset and course establishing a cause is difficult. At the University of California, Davis, Medical Center, about 20% of all new patients at the allergy and immunology clinic complain of a food allergy. In a handful of these individuals, the causal connection between trigger and symptom is obvious, because the time between ingestion of the offending food and the appearance of symptoms is measured in minutes. In the remaining 80% of cases, however, the history of the problem is confusing, and the cause unclear or uncertain with physician and patient having little to go on to establish a clear-cut diagnosis.

Bobby, 11, was referred to the clinic because of a puzzling history of recurring hives. Approximately three times a year, without warning, Bobby would break out with severe, itchy hives all over his body. He and his parents are absolutely convinced that food is responsible. Because the episodes occur irregularly, Bobby's recollection of what he has eaten is not particularly dependable, and he is often unable to remember anything unusual that he has eaten. Although there is no clear link between his hives and something specific he has eaten, his parents and he stubbornly hold to the view that food is doing the damage.

The doctors who examined Bobby are in a dilemma. They know he has hives because they can see the wheals all over his body. However, because the hives turn up so irregularly and are not accompanied by any obvious inciting factors, they are in the dark regarding the causes. Bobby and his parents want the clinic to run skin tests to nail down the food that is responsible for his troubles and refuse to accept the argument that there are no reliable, accurate ways of testing for Bobby's alleged food allergy. However, there are a number of reasons why this statement is true.

Food is such a complex mix of materials and undergoes so many chemical changes during its production, preservation, storage, preparation, and digestion that tens of thousands of combinations of what represents the substance to be tested are possible. Thus, as pointed out in Chapter 10, the skin test, the dependable mainstay for identifying respiratory allergens, is not especially effective when it comes to identifying food allergens. (Most allergists will not order skin tests for food allergies or insensitivities; the ones who do do so with great misgivings and have little reason to hope that the tests will point to a single clear-cut cause.)

There are other tests to determine if an allergic reaction is present in the body when the symptoms show; these blood tests, called RAST or FAST, are not designed to pin down the cause of a reaction; they simply indicate whether the reaction, whatever it is, has produced IgE antibodies. Also, these tests, too, yield unpredictable and sometimes confusing results. In small children, for example, researchers have found IgE antibodies not only in children allergic to milk, but also in those who do not have a milk allergy. Worse, they have detected no antibodies in children who have what seems to be a clear-cut history of milk allergy.

Some physicians also offer cytotoxic or sublingual (under the tongue) tests. Cytotoxic testing has been studied carefully and found to be devoid of any scientific merit; sublingual testing has also been the subject of several extensive reviews that question the procedure's utility. If your doctor recommends such testing, we recommend that you consult another physician to get a second opinion.

To discover what food or foods are causing a reaction in your child, an elimination diet can help you. What such a diet does is to start out by limiting the child to a few foods that are almost never responsible for reactions. If the symptoms persist, then food is probably not responsible for them. However, if the child gets better, then, at regular intervals, additional foods are added, and the reactions of the child are observed carefully as each new entrant appears. If the child shows a reaction, the food suspected of causing the reaction is dropped from the diet and then reintroduced after a waiting period. If the reaction occurs after the second exposure, there is good reason to believe that the offending food has been identified. A general elimination diet and specific diets free of mold, tyramine, salicylate, sulfite, cereals, and milk are given in Appendices A–D. If you suspect that food allergies are responsible for your child's allergic reaction, putting the youngster on an elimination diet may tell you what is causing the problem. However, it is well to note that the diet is extremely boring, and children (and adults, too) have a hard time adhering to it. You must stick to it religiously; that is the only way that it can be made to work. Beyond that, with the enormous range of foodstuffs and their variability, the diet may fail to turn up any suspects. An elimination diet can help in diagnosis, but it is a drawn-out and crude process, and there is always the chance that it may not pay off in the end.

If you have a clue or hunch concerning what is causing your child's hypersensitivity reaction, either because there is a fairly good circumstantial case linking fast-developing symptoms to a specific food or because you have followed an elimination diet, then to be sure that you do have the food responsible, your doctor may want to do a challenge test.

In conducting a challenge test, the doctor will put samples of the suspected food and something innocuous that looks exactly like it—a placebo—in capsules. The child will then take either the placebo or suspected agent on a number of occasions and will be observed closely to see if the reaction occurs. (Neither the child nor the person administering the capsules will know what is being administered; this "double-blind" procedure is a routine precaution to see that the results obtained are unaffected by the patient's or physician's subjective beliefs and feelings.)

In summary, the diagnosis of food allergy or hypersensitivity—identifying the agent or agents that cause the symptoms—can be a difficult and often unsuccessful enterprise. A direct, clear, and unmistakable link between trigger and symptoms occurs perhaps in one case in five; for the remaining cases, an elimination diet followed by a properly conducted challenge test is the most accurate way to diagnose the cause.

Allergy or Intolerance-Causing Agents

Almost anything taken by mouth can cause a reaction in some susceptible person. This infinite potential for mischief makes it difficult to pin down the exact cause of an individual allergic or hypersensitive intolerance reaction. There are, however, a number of foods or materials found in foods that are well-known for their ability to provoke reactions.

Foods that trigger allergic or hypersensitive reactions in significant numbers of children and the type of reaction they can cause are listed in Table 3.

In addition, other substances found in food are often responsible for hypersensitive or allergic reactions. Table 4 names some of the more common agents, where they are encountered, and the symptoms they can produce.

Food is a vital part of our life and a major element in all cultures, and there is an enormous and diverse range of materials we can eat. See to it that your children follow a balanced diet, one that includes entries from all of the major food groups. Vegetarian families or ones that restrict themselves to one or a limited number of food groups should consult with a clinical nutritionist. Clinical nutritionists are on college or university faculties, on hospital staffs, in government agencies, or in private practice. Generally speaking, they are extremely helpful and, by assessing your family's diet, can assure you that you are not doing yourself harm with your dietary habits.

In addition to what is ingested, there are a few conditions the child may have that give the appearance of food allergy or intolerance although they are really owing to organic problems. These include enzyme deficiencies and gastrointestinal tract diseases, notably gastric and duodenal ulcers, hiatal hernia, and inflammatory bowel disease. These causes are uncommon in youngsters, but they do turn up occasionally.

In young children, food intolerances or allergies are usually reflected in gastric complaints—colic, stomachache, constipation, diarrhea. Chapter 10 deals specifically with these symptoms, their incidence, causes, and treatment.

Fad Diets

Hardly a day goes by without the appearance of yet another miracle diet that promises to melt away pounds, restore vitality, recover lost youth, replace falling hair, remove wrinkles, or deal miraculously with some problem that bothers people.

Avoid these media-touted miracles. Most of them are unproven; some are dangerous; all make money for someone, and most of them go out of favor in a short time because they simply do not work. However, people crave to do the right thing for themselves or the world they inhabit, and get a good feeling by eating right. We cannot emphasize too strongly the risks of food faddism.

Anna, a teenaged activist and environmentalist, conscientiously refused to eat any animal products. A take-no-prisoners vegetarian, she is health-conscious and spends serious money buying dietary supplements at a health food store. She believes that although she restricts what she eats, she can remain

Table 3
Foods Causing Hypersensitive or Allergic Reactions
in Children and Their Reactions

Food	Most Common Reactions
Milk	Diarrhea, abdominal pain, hives, skin rash, wheezing
Eggs	Abdominal pain, hives, wheezing
Cereals (wheat especially)	Hives
Nuts	Hives, wheezing
Legumes (peanuts, soybeans)	Hives, wheezing
Shellfish	Hives, wheezing
Tomatoes	Diarrhea, abdominal pain, skin rash
Berries	Hives, wheezing
Citrus fruits	Diarrhea, skin rash
Melons	Itchy palate or eyes

healthy just by taking vitamins and other supplements more or less indiscriminately. She has no clue regarding what she is eating or how it fits into a comprehensive, healthy diet; she simply believes the hype on the labels. However, after a year of this regimen, she developed diarrhea and a wide-ranging rash along with a nagging cold she could not seem to shake. She finally went to see her doctor, who was concerned that she had lost 25 pounds in the 9 months since her last visit. The doctor went over the diet that she followed, noting that it consisted mainly of a long list of herbs and supplements, including algae and seaweed, eked out with a variety of dried, processed fruits, and vegetables. The physician referred Anna to a clinical nutritionist who took a health history and immediately concluded that she probably was zinc-deficient. The nutritionist ran a zinc test, found that Anna's level stood at less than half of normal. She prescribed some zinc tablets, strongly encouraged Anna to change her diet, and worked out a balanced vegetarian diet with her. Within a week Anna felt much better and her skin was healing nicely.

A Special Word About Latex Allergy

Allergy to latex is discussed later in this book. Latex is found in a large variety of materials containing rubber, including balloons, condoms, and latex gloves. Latex allergy can be severe and even life-threatening. The reason for the special discussions about latex in this chapter on food allergy is very simple. Some people who are allergic to latex are also allergic to kiwi, bananas, avocado, melon, and Brazil nuts. We do not know why this cross-reaction exists, but it can be serious.

Treatment of Food Allergy or Hypersensitivity

To prevent the recurrence of symptoms brought on by a food allergy or intolerance, the obvious tactic is to avoid ingesting the substance respon-

Table 4
Nonfood Substances Causing Hypersensitivity Reactions,
Where They are Found, and the Reactions They Cause

Causal Agent	Found In	Most Common Reactions
Mold	Cheeses, fermented meats, fermented beverages like beer, dried fruits, yogurt	Wheezing
Antibiotics (bacitracin, penicillin, tetracycline)	Meats, poultry, milk	Hives, skin rash, wheezing
Insect residue	Spices	Diarrhea, abdominal pain, hives
Herbicides, pesticides	Fruits, vegetables	Skin rash
Preservatives		
Sulfiting agents	Dried foods	Wheezing, bloating
Nitrates and nitroids	Preserved meats	Diarrhea, abdominal pain wheezing
Sodium benzoate and benzoic acid	Ketchup, pickles	Diarrhea, abdominal pain, wheezing
Sodium proprionate	Stored meats and fish; many breads	Diarrhea, abdominal pain
BHA and BHT (butylated hydrox amerole and butylated hydroxytoluene)	Many dried foods such as dry cereals	Diarrhea, abdominal pain
Food coloring		
Tartrazine (yellow food dye #5)	Taco, potato, or other chips, dry cereals, some medications; ubiquitous	Wheezing
Flavor "enhancers" and sweeteners		Diarrhea, abdominal pain
Monosodium glutamate (MSG)	Chinese or Japanese restaurant or packaged foods; other prepared foods	Diarrhea, abdominal, pain, sweating, rapid heart rate
Texturing Agents		a
Enzymes		a
Bleaches		a
Other chemicals		a
Bacteria and bacterial toxins		a

aThe number of reactions is too few to categorize and not completely documented.

sible. Where a food or foods are implicated, this means not eating that food or, often, other foods that belong to the same family as the one found to be responsible. (Food family groupings are given in Appendix B.)

Where chemicals or other additives or contaminants are concerned, avoiding the offending substance may be a bit more difficult. Table 4 lists the problems caused by such agents. If the agents causing the reaction are additives, be especially attentive to content labels. The major sources of trouble are sulfiting agents that are used as preservatives, and tartrazine, food dye #5. Appendices D-4 and D-5 name some of the more common places where these additives are found.

A general procedure to follow in identifying foods or food additives or contaminants responsible for allergic or hypersensitive reactions is sketched in Fig. 5, page 79. Observing the steps and precautions spelled within the figure should enable you to keep your child from harm.

Medications, especially over-the-counter drugs, should not be used to treat food intolerances unless approved by your doctor.

Too Much of a Good Thing

We have encountered food-linked complications in significant numbers of allergic children.

First, some youngsters have been kept needlessly sedentary or inactive with their allergies being given as the reason. One result of this enforced inactivity has been overweight or, in some instances, obese youngsters. In allergic children, this carries serious side effects. It inhibits developing the ability to resist or fight off some complaints like asthma, and it is associated with higher levels of vulnerability to allergy-linked complaints, like chronic earache.

Second, there is a strong tendency for parents to think of a robust appetite as a sign of good health. Accordingly, they ply sick children with food treats and delicacies, apparently in the belief that if they see the child eating heartily, he or she is on the road to health and well-being. Food is not a medicine; a sound, sensible diet is necessary to good health, but merely consuming food will not cure anything. Forget folk sayings like "Feed a cold and starve a fever," or vice versa.

We have recently seen an upsetting increase in the number of allergic children we have treated who also show symptoms of bulimia, a psychologically linked disorder marked by a morbidly increased appetite associated with recurrent vomiting. We have the sense that this pattern of eating behavior sometimes originates with the parents' excessive concern over the underlying allergic condition—usually asthma—and their unconscious attempt to treat it with excessive amounts of food.

5

Colds and Respiratory Infections

Colds are as much a part of childhood as Christmas or "Sesame Street." Between the ages of 2 and 4, a child typically experiences 10 or more colds per year. Children in daycare or those from large families are especially prone to respiratory infections.

It is misleading to use the word "cold" because cold symptoms take many forms and can be produced by any of a huge list of viruses. The four major types of viruses known to produce upper respiratory diseases are respiratory syncytial virus, rhinovirus, parainfluenza, and influenza. Respiratory syncytial virus infections occur only in infants; there are nearly 100 different subtypes of rhinovirus, and numerous versions of parainfluenza and influenza that can infect individuals of any age. There is no vaccine to protect children from any of these infections despite the billions of dollars poured into research seeking cures for viruses.

Because of their numbers alone, it is impossible to develop immunity to all viral respiratory infections; in fact, recent evidence suggests that immunity to certain viruses is only temporary, and people can be reinfected repeatedly by the same virus.

These four major kinds of viruses interest us because they have all been shown to make allergies, particularly asthma, worse. For nonallergic children, colds and other routine respiratory infections are benign, clearing up on their own in a few days' time. For the allergic youngster, however, special thought and attention need to go into avoiding and preventing colds and respiratory infections.

Prevention of Colds and Respiratory Infections

Resistance to colds depends on many factors. In fact, one of the mysteries of medicine is why two people so very much alike in other respects respond so differently to respiratory infections.

> Jack and Jerry live on the same block. They were both born in February of 1981 and are now 16 years old. Jack hardly ever seems to get sick; Jerry, on the other hand, seems to have caught every cold that has ever shown up in the neighborhood and kept it longer than anyone else. Why?

"Why?" is a good question and one we cannot completely answer. Every reader knows that we cannot prevent or treat the common cold. However, there are steps we can take that affect how we develop infections. Inadequate nutrition, psychological stress, poor personal hygiene, lack of sleep or fatigue, recurrent diseases of the lung—all seem to be associated with more frequent respiratory infections.

The Importance of Good Nutrition

Americans have become a nation of junk food junkies. We eat nutritionally bankrupt breakfast cereals loaded with sugar and preservatives, and devoid of essential fiber, minerals, and vitamins. We have fatty fast food lunches that are about as well-balanced nutritionally as the styrofoam containers they come in. We eat too few vegetables, too many frozen and not enough fresh. We binge eat and drink. It is no accident that a significant percentage of our population have nutritionally associated lipid disorders in their blood—high cholesterol in other words. A number of surveys have shown that many schoolchildren have insufficient levels of zinc in their bodies, lack iron and other critical minerals and vitamins, and are anywhere from overweight to obese. These children can be regarded as "nutritionally-at-risk."

Following a well-balanced nutritional program is not necessarily going to prevent colds, but the person who is malnourished or not eating the "right stuff" is more likely to have common colds, and they will hang on longer than they do in people who eat properly. There are more diets than there are catalogs at Christmas, and we cannot even begin to evaluate and critique them. However, we can point out one good take-home lesson. Hospital dietitians as a group are friendly and helpful. No matter how small or big the hospital, you will find that the registered dietitian is a source of good, free information on dietary and nutritional questions.

For those with access to the internet, a really good web site is: http://www.eatright.org/readlist.html. This site contains a long list of textbooks and free information in the consumer market, including materials from the U.S. Department of Agriculture and American College of Pediatrics. For those people who want to read something, a good start is *Eating the Alphabet* by Lois Ehlert, Harcout Brace Jovanovich Publishing, 1989. There is also a consumer nutrition hotline at 800-366-1655 that presents timely food and nutrition messages in English or Spanish.

Psychological Stress

We do not know why individuals under physical or emotional stress are more likely to develop illnesses. A large number of experimental studies in animals reveal that under stress, infection occurs more readily; stress in humans is also associated with an increased incidence of injury or illness. We talk about stress and how to manage it in Chapter 22.

Hygiene and General Health Habits

Most people wrongly believe that colds are spread by being coughed or sneezed on by a person already infected. Certainly being coughed or sneezed on is not likely to promote good health nor good relationships for that matter. However, the data now show that colds are mainly transmitted by hand contact—shaking hands with an infected person, using communal towels, and so on. Since most cold-carrying viruses are passed along without the person realizing he or she is being infected, unceasing preventive strategies must be followed in order to reduce the likelihood of contracting a cold. Here are some steps your children (and you) can take to cut the number and severity of colds.

1. Practice good health habits: get plenty of sleep, eat properly.
2. Keep in good physical shape: exercise regularly, watch the weight.
3. Avoid contact with people who are coughing or sneezing.
4. Do not get overheated; avoid drafts.
5. Drink plenty of fluids (at least 1 quart daily).
6. Where indicated get flu or pneumovax shots.
7. Wash hands with soap frequently during the day and always after using the bathroom and before meals; keep hands away from the nose, eyes and mouth.
8. Do not share eating utensils or glassware; avoid public drinking fountains.
9. Have individual towels; do not use communal towels.
10. If you have a cough or cold, cover the mouth when sneezing or coughing.

Recurrent or Chronic Lung Diseases

Other conditions contribute to catching colds, including underlying pre-existing illness. Children with cystic fibrosis (CF), a serious respiratory disease, have severe recurrent respiratory infections that often become life-threatening. CF children produce too much thick mucus; the mucus clogs the airways, and bouts of pneumonia often follow. Additionally, children with histories of recurrent pneumonias or those who have congenital defects that impair normal cleansing of the lung—those born with abnormal airways, for example—are also more likely to have their colds turn serious. Children with asthma also seem to have more respiratory infections, and they seem to grow more severe as the child ages.

As well as being dangerous in other ways, smoking tobacco or illicit drugs make the user more vulnerable to respiratory infections. Parents who allow their children to smoke tobacco or dope are at best irresponsible and certainly negligent. Also exposure to second-hand smoke spells bad news for asthmatic children.

> Ellen seems to be sick all the time; she missed 10 days of school in November alone. Her mother thinks she does everything right. Ellen dresses well, eats balanced meals, gets a full night's sleep, and yet has recurrent colds and sinus infections. Ellen's doctor has a hard time getting the mother to understand that part of the problem is the tobacco smoke in the house. Both parents each smoke a pack of cigaretts per day.

Tobacco smoke can go a long way toward making a child sick and for the encore it kills.

6

Airborne Allergens

Airborne substances are the single most common cause of allergic reactions. In addition to provoking respiratory allergic symptoms in children—mainly seasonal or chronic hay fever or asthma—they may intensify complaints like eczema, and they are often linked to other problems, such as chronic earache, itchy, teary eyes, and gastrointestinal difficulties. The symptoms follow a period of sensitization and are uncommon in children before the age of 4.

The most important airborne allergens are:

Plant pollens;
Molds;
Dust, including mites and cockroaches;
Animal dander;
Smoke (especially tobacco smoke);
Pollutants (industrial or vehicular); and
Other airborne particles (insect parts, soaps, detergents, and other household cleaning materials, chemicals).

Plant Pollens

Plants give off pollen as part of their reproductive cycle. The tiny pollen spores (thousands of them could comfortably occupy the head of a pin) invade the respiratory passages and, in the susceptible child, bring on the symptoms of hay fever.

You can broadly determine if plants are responsible for your child's distress by noting whether or not the symptoms are seasonal—and, if so, during what season they occur. If they turn up only during the early spring, chances are good that pollens are at fault—pollens from trees in particular. If they appear late in spring or during the summer, grasses or weeds are more likely

Table 5
Sources of Airborne Molds or Fungi

Indoor	Outdoor
Damp basements or crawl spaces	Leaf or plant surfaces (grasses, hay, or
Bathrooms and showers	wheat-growing areas especially)
Window frames	Decomposing (decaying) plant materials
Utility rooms	
House plants	
Rubber or foam pillows	
Vaporizing, humidifying,	
or air-conditioning equipment	

to be implicated. (Appendix E gives the times when various kinds of pollens become airborne throughout the United States.)

Not all plants give off allergy-producing pollens. Goldenrod, for one example, once drew the blame for the hay fever that turns up in the late summer and early fall in the eastern and midwestern United States; ragweed, the real culprit, has the same blooming cycle but did not harvest the blame initially because it does not flower as showily as goldenrod.

Chapter 12 also tells how to control hay fever symptoms. When they are the result of pollen, avoiding or minimizing contact with the offending substance is the most effective tactic although difficult to carry out in practice. Air-filtering devices are extremely helpful in cleaning out pollen. Your physician or HMO can suggest what kind of device to use, and Appendix F sketches tactics you can use to locate suppliers.

Molds and Fungi

Breathing in spores from mold or fungi is another important cause of chronic hay fever or asthma in susceptible and sensitized youngsters. Molds occur both indoors and out-of-doors, and a large number of them are capable of triggering symptoms. Establishing that they are at fault and identifying the one or ones responsible for symptoms is a difficult and imprecise business, because their sheer numbers make developing a comprehensive battery of tests next to impossible.

Fungi and molds thrive under warm, moist conditions. Consequently they and the symptoms they cause are more likely to flourish during the warm, more humid seasons of the year. Major indoor and outdoor sources of mold and fungi are listed in Table 5.

Chapter 12 goes into control procedures for molds and fungi. Scrupulous cleanliness is important; in addition, if the child's allergic symptoms are

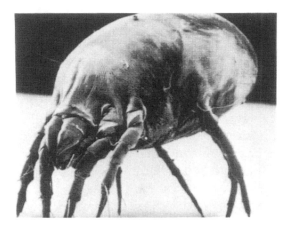

Fig. 2. Dust mite.

chronic and resist treatment, air purification devices and hypoallergenic decor in the bedroom of the affected person will help.

Dust

Dust, inside or out-of-doors, causes allergic reactions—usually perennial allergic rhinitis—in some youngsters. Parents cannot do much about outdoor dust except try to limit the child's exposure to it. House dust is a different and somewhat more manageable nuisance.

Although house dust contains a little bit of everything, its single most important component insofar as allergic youngsters are concerned is the dust mite.

Dust mites, pyroglyphidae, come in four species. Microscopic in size, they are the ingredient in house dust mainly responsible for dust allergy. Figure 2 shows one of the culprits, greatly enlarged. They thrive in warm, humid conditions and their bodies and fecal pellets, when inhaled, trigger hay fever-like symptoms in susceptible individuals.

The dust mite lives in fabrics—carpeting, upholstery, cloth wall hangings, curtains and drapes, mattresses, blankets.

Cleanliness—particularly of the bedroom—is the key to control of allergies triggered by house dust mites. In addition to the general control measures given in Chapter 12, here are some specific things you can do to get rid of dust—and dust mites.

1. Use plastic shades or blinds instead of curtains and drapes.
2. Remove rugs, fabric wall hangings, and overstuffed furniture. Replace with plain wood or plastic.
3. Keep clothes in a closet. Keep the closet door shut.

4. Clean every other day, using a damp cloth or mop to pick up dust. Do not sweep or vacuum. Pay special attention to dust-catchers like radios, TVs, or other electronic gear, books, and bureau drawers.
5. Beware of toys, especially plush or stuffed dolls. If there are any (current fashion seems to call for the child's bed to be buried under a mound of them) send them away on a long visit.
6. Use hypoallergenic bed clothes (mattress and pillow cover, sheet, blanket), if necessary.
7. Control temperature and humidity with a room air conditioner. (Keeping the relative humidity at less than 50% will kill the pests.)
8. Install an air cleaner, if necessary.
9. Wash pillow covers and bedsheets in hot water (150°F) once a week.

Animal Dander

Animals—their dander, actually sloughed off skin, fur, feathers—spell misery for many allergic children. By animals, we mean not only cats and dogs—horses, rabbits, hamsters, mice, rats, and birds can provoke the chronic hay fever symptoms shown by vulnerable people.

It is not just the animals themselves—their food or water dishes can harbor mold or fungi, they carry parasites that can be troublesome in their own right, bird droppings dried and dispersed are known to cause serious lung disorders, and even some pet food ingredients can trigger a reaction. What appears to do the most damage, however, is breathing in dried dead skin cells, whatever the species, and dried saliva (from cats cleaning themselves). The make of animal (small, large, shorthair, longhair) seems unimportant; it is not the hair, but what is under it that mainly causes the problem.

The safest pet for an allergic child is a Pet Rock. (Even fish tanks sprout mold that can provoke sniffling or wheezing). For allergic children, the most prudent course is to keep no pets at all, to avoid contact with other people's pets, and to take preventive measures when going into a situation where animals were or are present. Medications that can block reactions to animal dander or other animal-induced allergies and strategies for using them are given in Chapter 12.

Smoke

Smoke frequently causes asthmatic symptoms—wheezing and shortness of breath. Any type of smoke can be responsible, but the most common villains are tobacco smoke, smoke from wood-burning stoves or fireplaces, and candles.

If your child is sensitive to smoke, the obvious course to follow is to see to it that there is as little contact with it as possible.

Cigarette smoke is the major source of trouble, and if the child is bothered by it, house and automobile should be declared smoke-free zones—

easier said than done. (Even if children are not sensitive to cigarette smoke, they should be spared exposure to it; the damage to lungs from ambient tobacco smoke extends far beyond triggering wheezing.)

Quitting smoking when as powerfully addictive a drug as nicotine is involved is a severe test of fortitude and will. However, millions of Americans, recognizing the mortal danger of the habit, have been able to shake it. If you have not succeeded, now may be the time for the effort that will see you win through; your HMO or the local American Lung Association offers information about quitting smoking.

If wood smoke associated with home heating represents a problem for your youngster, you can at least minimize the problem by ensuring that the stove is tight and well vented to the outside. Clean, unobstructed stove pipes and an adequate draught ought to ensure that the house itself is largely smoke-free.

Candles or incense, since they are burned largely for ambiance or decor, can be readily discarded. If the birthday cake has to have a candle, keep it to one. The symbolism will be preserved, and more importantly, so will the health and well-being of the child.

Pollutants

Industrial and vehicular emissions are responsible for respiratory problems, too. They are more likely to be a significant factor in urban, industrialized settings—most of the major cities in the United States have occasional to near-permanent periods of moderate to severe air pollution. Even Denver, once a haven for asthma sufferers, has a perennial smog problem.

Strategies to follow in coping with air pollution are spelled out in Chapter 11.

Other Airborne Allergens

Robby, 6, loves to go to the supermarket with his mom. She is understandably reluctant to have him along, partly because almost any 6-year-old is a loose cannon in a supermarket, and partly because Robby always goes into a violent fit of sneezing and coughing when they pass down the aisle where the soaps and detergents are shelved.

The environment has been invaded by literally thousands of chemicals, many of which can become airborne and cause respiratory symptoms of one kind or another. Most airborne chemicals that are a problem emit pungent odors. Thus, it is more often an irritant effect than an allergy. Clearly we have much to learn about the role of chemicals in allergies. Until we do, parents of children troubled by chemicals will have to learn how to deal with the symptoms they produce through trial and error—possibly with some help from the doctor.

7

Weather, Climate, and Exercise

In addition to the myriad substances that can cause allergic reactions, many allergic children also have to contend with the fact that the mere accident of being or doing can provoke or worsen their symptoms. Extremes of heat or cold, the seasons of the year, and the level of activity of your child can and often do have a bearing on allergic symptoms.

Cold

Exposure to cold in and of itself can trigger or worsen asthma or hives directly. Wearing wool, leather, fur, or down garments to keep warm can also start a child wheezing or itching with eczema or contact dermatitis. Cold air is a major problem for asthmatics. Sometimes just the act of stepping outside on a cold day is enough to induce bronchospasm.

Ben, 10, has had moderate asthma since he was 2. He lives in a small town near Buffalo, New York, which is justly renowned for its harsh winters. One extremely cold, snowy, and windy Sunday, he, his parents, and younger brother are returning home from church. The car hits an icy patch and slides off the road into the ditch. His mother and brother are slightly shaken up. The father stays to minister to them and instructs Ben to run to a nearby house for help. The house is only about 300 yards away, but Ben, as soon as he gets out into the frigid gale, starts wheezing. His wheezing seems to get worse with each step he takes, and he can barely manage to struggle to the house. By this time, his breathing is so bad that when his knock is answered, he is unable to say what the trouble is and, almost in shock, can only point outside and gasp "Help!" The householder immediately senses the trouble, has Ben go into the warm house, and telephones for help to go to the accident scene.

This wheezing problem can be controlled by adopting tactics that warm the air before it gets to the airways—filtering it through a scarf or ski mask, for example.

Hives can be caused by many physical, environmental factors—see Chapter 14 for the various causes. Cold-induced urticaria (hives) is especially important, because it is quite common and can become so severe that its victims literally have to stay bundled up all winter. Any lapse will result in children developing hives and enduring the maddening itching that accompanies them. Indeed, the symptoms can become more generalized, and cause severe shortness of breath or even a shock reaction.

> Tom has had cold-induced urticaria for 3 years. He is now 12 and enjoying summer camp—or at least he was until he jumped into the lake. The water felt cold as soon as he hit it, and he knew that he should not have done it. Within seconds, his body started to swell and itch and he got very, very short of breath. That was the last thing he remembered. His camp counselor said he was lucky to be alive and only survived because it happened to be the day of the doctor's weekly visit to the camp. His prompt and effective action saved Tom's life.

Tom's near-fatal reaction is rare, but when a reaction like this does occur, sudden immersion in water is often responsible. To control cold-induced hives, see to it that your child dresses appropriately and avoids sudden exposure to cold air or water.

Heat

Extreme heat can be particularly troublesome for children with eczema. These children are warned to keep from sweating and overheating—warnings that are difficult, if not impossible to enforce. However, the plain fact is that excessive heat dries the skin and causes it to crack and itch; it also induces sweating, which can make the skin irritable, especially where it comes into contact with clothing. Eczema flourishes under these conditions and should be managed along the lines sketched in Chapter 13.

Heat and Cold

Some children suffer chronically from a condition known as vasomotor rhinitis. Although this is not an allergic complaint, youngsters with it have stuffy noses throughout the year, and the snuffles are made worse by breathing in air that shows any significant extreme in temperature. Going out into the cold will start the nasal faucet running; even sniffing a hot mug of soup can be troublesome. (Vasomotor rhinitis is discussed in Chapter 12.)

Oftentimes a humidifier is prescribed as a remedy for vasomotor rhinitis. This approach is usually ineffective, and as we point out in Chapter 20, can put the child at risk to mold allergies if the device is carelessly or improperly maintained. About the only thing a parent can do when confronting this problem is to teach the child to carry a good supply of tissues and to blot—not blow—the flow. (Blowing has the tendency to force mucus into the sinus cavities and is associated with sinus infections.)

Barometric Pressure and Humidity

Changes in barometric pressure and humidity level, along with the temperature, affect asthmatics. Asthma is inversely related to all three of these features of climate, that is, the lower the humidity, temperature, or barometric pressure, the greater the likelihood of bronchospasm. Since, as Charles Warner once observed, "Everybody talks about the weather but nobody does anything about it," your strategy here is to do what you can to maintain a comfortable temperature and a good level of relative humidity—60–70%—indoors. (Keeping to this standard should also cut the risk of eczema, if that is also a possibility, and will reduce energy costs as well.)

The susceptibility of asthmatics to low humidity and cold is one reason we recommend swimming. Exercise or activity done in moist, warm conditions does not seem to precipitate wheezing.

The Seasons

As any hay fever sufferer knows, a year has two seasons—hay fever time and the rest of the year.

Depending on the plants responsible, hay fever can turn up at any time during the growing season.

Since parents cannot stop the plants from growing or children from playing outside, they are left to take preventive and control measures that are spelled out in Chapter 12. The main thing is to be aware of when the problem is due to turn up and to get ready for it beforehand.

Activity and Exercise

Exercise or activity, in itself, can induce asthma. It can also provoke hives and cause eczema to appear or worsen.

With asthma, the type of exercise and the conditions under which it is done have an important bearing on events. Sustained exertion under dry or cold weather conditions will almost certainly bring on wheezing. Asthmatics should avoid jogging or distance running; swimming, as we have already noted, working with weights or weight apparatus, or other short-burst activities ordinarily carry no significant consequences.

Medicating appropriately will usually forestall exercise-induced asthma. As described later, even Olympic gold-medalists have had exercise-induced asthma. However, it is important to note that allergists and chest physicians are becoming increasingly aware of two other aspects of exercise-induced asthma. The first of these is a delayed response where the bronchospasm does not occur until several hours after the exercise is over. The reason for this is unknown, but the existence of the phenomenon reminds us of the need for asthmatics to be judicious about exercise—to stick to what is appropriate for them and to be scrupulous about following preventive measures.

The second complication is that exercise can have a synergistic or additive impact on asthmatic children. Thus, if your child's chest is already tight from a cold or allergic asthma, exercise-induced bronchospasm can make matters worse, even to the point of forcing a trip to the emergency room.

Finally, there is a disease known as exercise-induced anaphylaxis (EIA). EIA is a seldom-encountered condition that occurs with exercise. A small number of children are so bothered by exercise that anaphylaxis—shock and vascular collapse, an extremely dangerous and sometimes lethal condition—can follow exertion. The condition is extremely rare, but its existence underscores the fact that what is simple fun to most can add up to tragedy for an unfortunate few.

Part Three

The Common Allergic Diseases,

Why Children Develop Them, and The Steps You, The Parent, Can Take To Diagnose, Treat, Control, and Avoid Their Symptoms

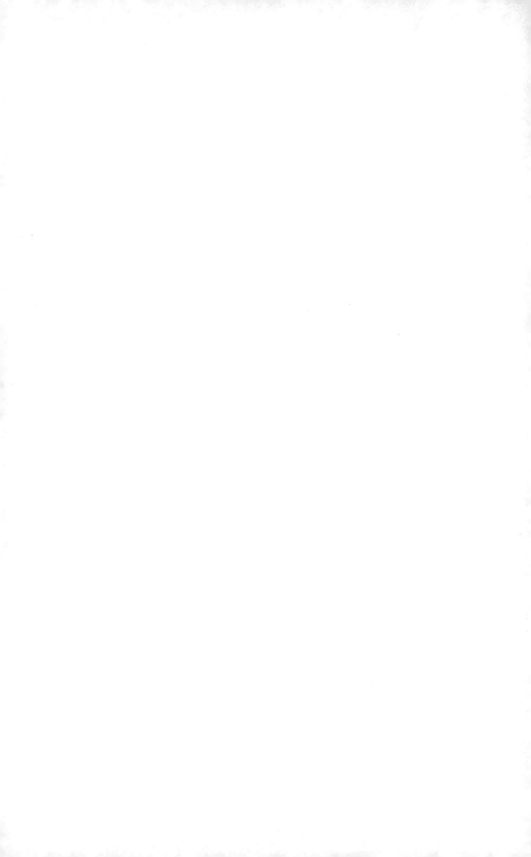

8

Skin Irritants

Skin irritation—dermatitis—is commonplace; almost all children show various kinds of skin rashes or outbreaks as they grow up. Rashes are the most common reason for new mothers to bring their babies to the pediatrician. Rashes may have any of a number of causes and may take any of a variety of forms. The most common ones are those arising from contact with one of the literally thousands of substances capable of causing the skin to erupt. A red rash, blisters, or hive-like wheals—all with or without itching—may be the result.

There are different classes of agents responsible for skin outbreaks in children. The age of the child has a good deal to do with which one is responsible and the form the symptoms take. The interrelationships between the age of the child and the nature, location, cause, and character of skin problems are described fully in Chapter 17.

In the great majority of cases, contact dermatitis is not an allergic reaction, even though there is a well-exercised tendency to label it as such.

Joel, a high school student and a computer whiz helps out in the family business. He spends most of one weekend working with his father to set up a new accounts receivable and billing system. That Sunday evening he notices that his hands and face have become quite inflamed, red, tender, and itchy. He and his folks are mystified by this development until they review the weekend's activities and recall that Joel has spent most of that time sorting through stacks of pressure-sensitive invoice copies. Joel is simply hypersensitive to one or another of the chemicals with which the forms are impregnated, although he and his folks like to say that he is allergic to them.

During earlier and simpler times, dermatitis did not represent as much of a problem as it does today. Although parents have always had diaper rash or poison oak to contend with, what makes the problem larger, more baffling, and more difficult to manage is the accelerating invasion of all parts of the environment by chemicals. These substances, whose aim is to make life easier, often have the effect of rendering it exactly the opposite. Hardly a day passes without a new—or "improved"—household product being thrown on the market. Cleaning agents, waxes, polishes, solvents, stain preventives, stain removers, and a bewildering variety of other household products keep turning up.

These manufactured substances are found everywhere—at home or school, in the workplace, in the automobile. They occur in fabrics, leathers, jewelry, and cosmetics; they are components of printer's ink, glue, and toys; ironically, they are even found in some topical medications.

In addition to this constantly growing number of man-made irritants is the almost limitless number of naturally occurring ones.

Carla, 6, accompanies her mother to the library one fine morning in early spring. While her mother is inside, Carla amuses herself by climbing a low-branching olive tree in the library's backyard. Books found and checked out, Carla's mom collects Carla and sets off to run the rest of the morning's errands. They do not get completed, though. In about 30 minutes, Carla develops an itch followed by a case of hives involving much of her body and has to be rushed home. Her reaction to the heavy pollen and sap of the blooming tree clears rapidly, however. By evening she is able to resume her outdoor play.

The beneficial effects of the manufactured, fabricated products are trumpeted insistently—some of the miracles claimed for them may even be true—but their negative impact on the health and well-being of some users gets the silent treatment. Whether the product is capable of causing an itch or a rash in the user is a nuisance question to the manufacturer. It probably can—almost anything will, given a susceptible individual—but looking for and then issuing a warning about possible harmful side effects would run costs up and harm sales. Quite flatly, many manufacturers show little or no concern over seeing to it that their products do not represent a hazard to the consumer.

Given this "let the buyer beware" attitude, what steps can you take to protect your youngsters from developing skin irritations? Here are some tactics you can follow that will at least reduce the risk or minimize the consequences of coming into contact with dermatitis-causing substances.

1. Be familiar with the forms the most common skin irritations take and their causes.
2. When a rash develops, be especially attentive to where it occurs on the body.
3. Review the child's activities carefully to try to pin down a cause for the problem.

4. Apply first-aid measures that will relieve the rash and the itching or pain that usually accompanies it.
5. Help the child to recognize and avoid whatever is causing the symptoms.
6. Be alert to the possibility of a secondary infection developing; if one does, consult your physician at once.
7. Help the child deal constructively with the problem in a supportive, stress-free atmosphere. Keep in mind that the youngster does not want the problem, did not get it deliberately, is probably suffering acutely, and since it is not contagious, cannot give it to anyone else.
8. If the condition persists for more than a few days or shows signs of worsening, see your doctor.
9. Remember, most skin irritations are minor, short-lived, easily managed, and have no permanent adverse effects on either appearance or general health.

Drug stores are filled with over-the-counter creams, ointments, and gels that promise relief of skin conditions. Most are expensive and not worth the money. Some can even make matters worse.

Carla had a skin rash. Her mother picked up a bottle of Calamine lotion with Benadryl at the drug store. The lotion seemed to help the rash at first, but suddenly it took a turn for the worse. Carla's skin looked red and angry. A trip to the doctor convinced Carla and her mother that the culprit was the Benadryl in the Calamine lotion. Carla had become allergic to it.

Before using any over-the-counter drug for any condition, read the label and the directions carefully. Look for ingredients that trigger reactions in your youngsters, and read the fine print carefully, especially the sections that talk about negative reactions or possible side effects.

9

Insect Stings or Bites*

Incidence

Allergic or hypersensitive reactions to insect stings or bites are fairly common; just how common nobody knows. Individuals showing moderate to severe reactions to or developing secondary infections to stings or bites are among the more frequently seen patients in the doctor's office or clinic.

Usual Age of Onset

Almost everyone, on being stung or bitten by an insect, shows some sort of reaction, but its severity will vary greatly from person to person. Stings or bites causing more than slight temporary discomfort (slight, temporary discomfort is by far the typical experience) can and do occur at any age. As a general rule, however, the intensity of the reaction is directly tied to age or the number of prior exposures. Thus, individuals over 18 or ones who have had frequent encounters with the insect and have become sensitized to it are the ones most likely to show troublesome reactions. Infants or small children, although known on occasion to have serious reactions, are the least likely to come up with them.

Symptoms

After a child is bitten or stung by an insect, he or she will likely run to you complaining of symptoms in vague, general terms. Sometimes the child (and you) will be quite unaware that an insect is responsible for them.

There are literally thousands of different insects, and many of them sting or bite humans. Table 6 names and lists the symptoms associated with the small number of insects responsible for most of the bite or sting problems encountered in the United States.

*Inhaling dust or debris that contains insect matter—wings, hair, body material, waste—can also cause reactions. *See* Chapters 6 and 12 for information about airborne allergens and how to deal with them.

Table 6
Stinging and Biting Insects and the Symptoms They Cause

Stinging Insects	Sting site	Symptoms		
		Immediate	1–20 minutes	20+ minutes
Honey bee,[a] wasp,[a] hornet,[a] and yellow jacket[a]	Exposed parts of body	Sharp, intense pain	Wheal at sting , site inflammation	Local swelling, itching, inflammation
Fire ant[a,b]	Exposed parts of body	Sharp, intense, burning pain	Blister or blisters at sting site, inflammation	Local swelling, itching, inflammation

Biting insects	Bite site	Symptoms		
		Immediate	1–20 minutes	20+ minutes
Mosquito	Exposed parts of body	Brief, barely noticeable prick	Wheal and inflammation	Small, itchy lesion at site
Fly	Exposed parts of body	Sharp pain	Wheal and inflammation	Small, itchy lesion at site
Wheel bug[a]	Hands and arms	Sharp, intense pain	Swelling, inflammation	Swelling, itching, inflammation
Kissing bug[a]	Face, hands, arms, legs	None	Itching at bite site	Swelling, intense itching, inflammation
Bedbug[a]	Face, hands, arms, legs	None	Itching at bite site	Swelling, intense itching, inflammation
Chigger	Legs and feet	Sharp pain	Wheal and itching at bite site	Small, itchy lesion
Flea	Feet and legs	Slight prick	Itching at bite site	Small, itchy lesion
Crab louse	Pubic area	None	None	Itchy lesion develops after infestation
Head louse	Scalp	None	None	Itchy lesion develops after infestation
Gnat	Exposed parts of body	Pain	Itch, swelling, and pain	Swelling, inflammation
Scabies mite	Much of body	None	None	Itchy lesion develops after infestation

[a]In extremely sensitive persons, may produce any or all of the following symptoms; hives and intense itching over much of the body, feelings of faintness, swelling of mucus tissue in throat, wheezing and difficulty in breathing. If any of these symptoms occur, seek emergency help immediately!
[b]The fire ant is also capable of administering painful bites with its powerful jaws. The stings often form a circular pattern of small burn-like blisters around the bite site.

Habitats of Stinging and Biting Insects

Honey bees, wasps, hornets, and yellow jackets are found throughout the United States. The fire ant belongs to the same insect family as the bees, wasps, and so forth, but is confined to the 13 southeastern and Gulf coast states.

As for biting insects, mosquitoes, biting flies, bedbugs, lice, fleas, scabies mites, and ticks are also found throughout the United States. Chiggers live in the southeast and southwest; wheel bugs occupy the area south of New York state, west and south to Texas; kissing bugs are prevalent in the south, southwest, and along the Pacific coast.

First Aid and Home Treatment of Insect Stings and Bites

Figures 3 and 4 trace first aid and home treatment measures to follow for insect stings or bites. You will see that there is some overlap in the charts —pain, swelling, and itching, whatever the cause, call for similar remedies, *and* the need to seek emergency attention when reactions have the potential to become general or life-threatening applies to both stings and bites.

We have given the best and most up-to-date ways of treating stings or bites. There are literally scores of other remedies to be had, but there is little or no evidence that they are as sure and safe as the ones we have mentioned.

Avoiding Insect Stings and Bites

The first line of defense against insects that cause allergic or hypersensitive reactions is to stay away from them and keep them away from your child. Steps you can take to avoid or control these insect pests are spelled out below. For the sting-sensitive child, the best tactic is to teach the youngster to avoid contact with stinging insects. Take the following precautions:

1. Tell the child where the insects live and work, and how to stay away from hives, nests, and ant hills.
2. Keep the child's body covered when outdoors during the bug season—long sleeves, trousers, shoes, and socks. Avoid brightly colored garments or loose-fitting clothes or hairdos that might trap the insects and provoke a sting.
3. Outlaw the use of any scent (perfume, deodorant, cologne, powder, lipstick, and so on) when the child is in the vicinity of stinging insects.
4. Instruct the child to be careful about eating out of doors as some species are attracted to foods.
5. Do NOT have the sting-sensitive child do lawn mowing, hedge-trimming, or other gardening activities that put him or her at risk.
6. Do NOT permit the child to go barefoot out-of-doors.

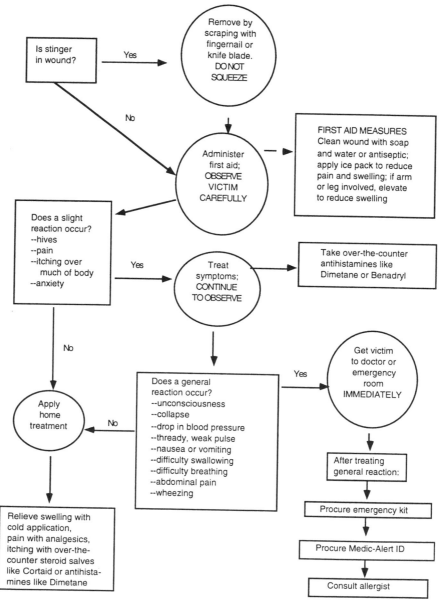

Fig. 3. First aid and home treatment for insect stings.

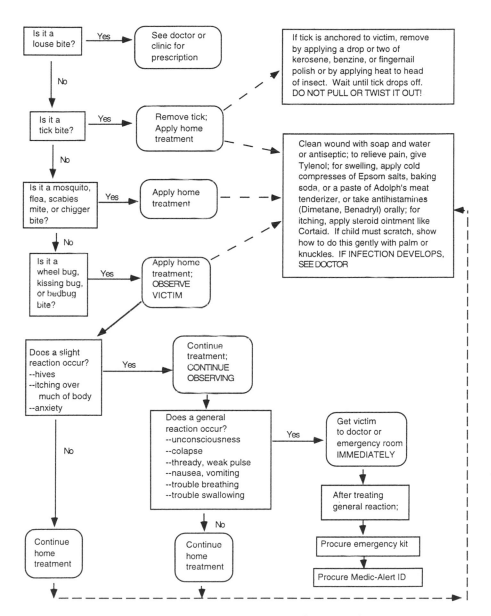

Fig. 4. First aid and home treatment for insect bites.

7. Instruct the child not to swat at or otherwise provoke an insect if it approaches or settles on the child. Show the child how to remain calm and slowly move out of harm's way. For the child who reacts to insect bites, Table 7 spells out steps that can be taken to avoid the various pests.

Controlling Stinging and Biting Insects

Stinging insects do not usually invade houses and tight screens are ordinarily all that is needed to keep the house secure. Fire ants, however, are attracted to food and, once inside, are difficult to eliminate. For eradication of fire ants and other stinging insects, consult state or federal Department of Agriculture offices for advice. If you decide on a program of eradication or choose to hire a pest control firm to carry it out, be especially alert to the fact that many pesticides carry substantial risks for humans and can cause serious damage, including compromise of the immune system.

Mosquitoes, flies, and kissing bugs can be screened out effectively. If fleas, lice, bedbugs, or kissing bugs do get established indoors, scrupulously cleaning the places they inhabit is usually enough to get rid of them in time. The Department of Agriculture has free pamphlets available that give detailed instructions on how to be rid of these nuisances. Wheel bugs, ticks, and chiggers are outdoor pests. They are difficult to control, although their numbers can be reduced to some extent by keeping vegetation trimmed, eliminating trash, and storing wood neatly—and away from the living quarters. As with stinging insects, the use of insecticides to get rid of biting insects should be done cautiously, as a last resort, and in strict compliance with the warnings that pesticide manufacturers are required to make known to users of their products.

Long-Term Treatment

If your youngster reacts severely to insect stings or bites you should take whatever precautions are necessary to prevent exposure. If the reaction is dangerous or life-threatening (rare, but known to happen in children), here are some additional steps you should take.

1. Obtain, learn how to use, and have an Epi-PEN available and ready for use at all times. (Your doctor will have to prescribe this kit, which contains antihistamines and a syringe preloaded with epinephrine.) This kit is much more user-friendly than its earlier version.
2. Have the child wear Medic-Alert identification, which will signal and specify the existence of a possible problem to anyone called on to administer emergency treatment. (Medic-Alert applications and information can be picked up in the doctor's office, clinic, or

Table 7
Avoiding Biting Insects

Tactic	Flies and mosquitoes[a]	Chiggers	Wheelbugs	Fleas	Ticks	Mites and lice
Use a repellent containing diethyl-toulamide.[a]	X	X			X	
Keep body covered—wear slacks, long sleeves, shoes, hat; avoid loose clothes or hairdos that could trap the insect	X	X	X		X	
Do not use scents or perfumes, lotions, cologne, deodorants, and so forth	X	X	X		X	
Insect-proof your pets				X	X	
Avoid contact with individuals infested with the pest						X

[a]Thiamine, vitamin B_1, which is available from health food stores or pharmacies, is thought to act as a mosquito repellent, but it can sometimes cause side effects—itching, hives, rash—and should be used with caution.

by writing the Medic-Alert Foundation, P.O. Box 1009, Turlock, CA 95381.)

3. A series of shots can desensitize your child to attacks by honey bees, wasps, hornets, yellow jackets, fire ants, or kissing bugs. The procedure—see Chapter 24 for details of how allergy shots work—almost always succeeds in reducing the severity of reactions to stings or bites dramatically. Talk to your physician or allergist about the possibility and appropriateness of desensitization for your child.

Complications

The two major complications associated with insect stings or bites are infections brought on by scratching and, in a few instances, anaphylactic or shock reactions brought on by the sting or bite.

To control itching, follow the treatment directions given in Figs. 3 and 4 on pp. 70 and 71; if infection does develop, consult your physician promptly.

Anaphylaxis occurs in individuals who are extremely susceptible to certain antigens. People have known since the time of the Pharaohs that bee stings could cause serious or even fatal reactions in some individuals. This anaphylactic or shock reaction can also be caused by injections—allergy shots are the most common cause, but penicillin, novocaine, and other medications and a wide list of foods are also capable of provoking this swift and dangerous response.

The anaphylactic reaction occurs rapidly—sometimes in a matter of seconds—and is marked by some or all of the following symptoms: massive outbreak of hives, swelling of mucous tissue, especially of the mouth and throat, wheezing or respiratory compromise, vascular collapse leading to a drop in blood pressure, faintness, or even loss of consciousness, nausea and vomiting, and feelings of anxiety, confusion, or dread.

This dangerous reaction requires immediate countermeasures. The standard treatment is to inject epinephrine, which reverses the drastic drop in blood pressure, and to administer antihistamines which counteract the massive histamine release, which is central to the problem.

A Special Note About Spiders

Many people fear or dread spiders and wrongly blame them for bites or stings actually delivered by other culprits. Only a couple of North American spiders—the Black Widow and Brown Recluse varieties—are dangerous. Their poisonous bites need to be treated immediately with antivenom serum, which will be available in a hospital emergency room or clinic. Note that children, because of their smaller body size and weight, are more likely to be endangered by bites of these spiders.

10

Gastrointestinal Complaints (Colic, Constipation, Diarrhea, and Stomachache)

At some time in their lives most children are likely to turn up with gastrointestinal problems—colic, constipation, diarrhea, or stomachache. In Table 8, we list these common conditions, their usual age of onset, their symptoms, and causes.

One especially prevalent problem in infants and young children is recurrent colic. Many mothers have had to suffer through the ordeal a colicky child presents. The theories about the cause of colic are legion; so are its remedies. This condition in young babies can be severe enough to cause extreme stress in the parents.

Tammy seemed like a normal baby until she was 8 weeks old. Then she started waking up virtually every night at 1:00 in the morning, irritable, restless, and crying. Nothing her parents did seemed to make her more comfortable. They discussed it with their pediatrician, who recommended eliminating milk from the diet. For 10 days immediately thereafter, Tammy's colic improved; then it started again exactly the same way as it was before. They tried everything and resorted to rocking the baby all night Finally, at 5 months of age, the colic disappeared, and Tammy's parents were at last able to get a decent night's sleep. Those 3 months were the worst ones they had ever experienced.

Milk allergy was strongly suspected in Tammy's case, but her experience did not indicate that milk was clearly to blame. Allergy to eggs in children is likewise common. Egg allergy, like milk allergy, can produce everything from eczema to wheezing to hives to abdominal pain.

Establishing the causes of these various gastrointestinal or stomach disorders in children is difficult, because they are manifold and obscure. For that reason, there is a well-established tendency to heap the blame for them on allergies—in particular, food allergies.

Table 8
Symptoms and Causes of Common Gastrointestinal
Complaints in Children According to Age

Symptoms	Age of onset	Probable condition	Cause
Abrupt, severe crying, clenched fists, drawing of knees to chest, tense and distended abdomen	Birth to 6 months	Colic	Not fully known; often associated with sensitivity to milk
Intermittent, recurring pain ranging from dull, cramping, or sharp, usually located near umbilicus	5–10 years	Chronic stomach-ache	Not fully known. Can arise from food allergy, constipation, migraine, irritable colon, psychological

Causes of Food Allergies and Intolerances in Children

Virtually any food or drink can trigger an adverse reaction in a susceptible child. The symptoms may grow out of a true allergic reaction and take any of the varied forms that characterize allergies—wheezing and shortness of breath, hives, angioedema (see Chapter 14 for definition of angioedema), eczema, hay fever, as well as the gastrointestinal complaints listed above, or sometimes the generalized, systemic life-threatening response of anaphylaxis. Male children, by a two-to-one margin, appear to be more prone to these allergic reactions, and susceptibility to them probably owes much to heredity.

A wide variety of foods, food colors, food preservatives, or pre-existing conditions in the individual can also produce symptoms that closely mimic allergic reactions and, in fact, account for most negative reactions to food (see Chapter 4). This mimicry makes specific diagnosis extremely difficult.

The diagnosis of a true allergy, as we noted in Chapter 1, requires the presence of the antibody IgE. This IgE binds onto special white cells known as basophils and/or mast cells, and under appropriate circumstances (such as your child eating the food he or she is sensitive or allergic to), these white cells release histamine and the other chemicals responsible for the allergic reaction. However, there are ways that foods and drugs can directly cause white cells to release histamine and chemicals without IgE involvement, and a large number of foods and drugs are capable of doing this. The best example of this is sensitivity to berries—strawberries, in particular—in children. Children sensitive to berries develop gastrointestinal problems, itching, hives—even full blown anaphylactic reactions. This sensitivity to berries often disappears as the child gets older. This may be owing to changes in the way that children and adults digest their food.

Sherry experienced her first bout of hives when she was 5, shortly after eating strawberries. She and her family quickly learned that berries would make her very sick and produce itchy skin bumps. Twenty years later, she tried a taste of fresh strawberry pie, and to her surprise and delight, found she was no longer sensitive.

Authorities believe that food allergy starts in infancy because a child's intestine is immature and allows for food to cross into the blood without complete digestion. This process can sensitize the child and pave the way for lifelong allergies. We suggest that some foods that are especially likely to induce food allergy—nuts, chocolate, and shellfish, among others—not be fed to children under 4 years of age. These foods are often linked to persistent and sometimes severe reactions.

Elise has been sensitive to peanuts all her life and has been very careful to avoid them. Recently, she developed hives all over her body after eating a handful of plain M & M's. She talked to her doctor, who called the manufacturer, who helpfully pointed out that the package label says: "This product may contain peanuts." Careful Elise let this one get by her.

The lessons here are that cross-contamination of foods is commonplace, and that Elise's problem might have been avoided if she had not been fed peanuts when she was young and more vulnerable.

Foods Associated with Gastrointestinal Symptoms in Children

The foods that appear on a list of the leading causes of food hypersensitivity (and gastrointestinal troubles) in children depend on the expert doing the listing. Although there is general agreement on the importance of cow's milk, eggs, shellfish, nuts, and wheat as provokers of reactions, the unanimity stops with them. Legumes (peanuts and soybeans) are frequently named, as are fish and mollusks. However, the authorities disagree on the role of tomatoes, chocolate, and citrus fruits, which are popularly identified as allergens, although strict laboratory experiments fail to support this charge. (Chocolate can make your child sick, but it is not borne out that the sickness is allergic.)

Allergic or hypersensitive gastrointestinal reactions in children can stem from a large assortment of additives or contaminants found in food.

The most important nonfood triggers of gastrointestinal problems in children are:

Gastrointestinal enzyme deficiencies in the child;
Antibiotic contaminants (bacitracin, penicillin, tetracycline) found in meats, poultry, or milk;
Insect residues found in spices;
Chemical food additives, including monosodium glutamate (MSG), metabisulfite, and tartrazine; and
Bacteria and bacterial toxins.

A Note on Milk and Enzyme Deficiencies in Children

Cow's milk is by far the most common reason for food sensitivity problems. This is not surprising considering the enormous quantity of milk consumed by children. This has been helped along by the earlier trend (now beginning to reverse) toward the use of bottled milk and milk-based formulas in lieu of breast-feeding. Thus, a much larger proportion of infants in the past two generations were bottle-fed—more than at any previous time in world history.

Cow's milk, whether whole, low-fat, or dry, contains many proteins. It also contains lactose, its principal sugar. A substantial percentage of blacks and Asians are born with a reduced amount of the enzyme lactase in their intestines. (This lack can also show up in young children of any ethnic origin.) Because they do not have an adequate amount of lactase to handle it, the milk sugar often passes undigested to their stomachs. Because it is passed undigested, it may undergo rapid transfer to the bowel, and lead to considerable bloating, stomach pain, diarrhea, and excessive gas. This is an intolerance rather than an allergy to milk. Lactase deficiency and the symptoms associated with it may also show up in people of any ethnic background who resume drinking milk after laying off of it for a period of weeks or months.

Identifying Food Intolerance

A strategy to follow in identifying the food (or the myriad of additives, contaminants, or other conditions) responsible for your child's hypersensitive reaction is sketched in Fig. 5. The figure outlines what is essentially a conservative, and minimally risky series of steps to follow. The key to successful attainment of the information you need is careful observance of an elimination diet. A general elimination diet together with the steps you will need to follow to see it through to a successful conclusion are presented in Appendix A. Following the procedures outlined in Fig. 5 and sticking faithfully to the elimination diet, if it is called for, should point to whatever is causing your child's food intolerance. The hardest part of the process may be getting the child to stay on the diet, which can be monotonous and boring.

First Aid and Home Treatment of Food Intolerance

Here we have the easiest part of the food hypersensitivity scenario—the means of avoiding a particular food are self-evident. *Avoid means avoid!* so long as you exercise a certain amount of vigilance and caution, you and your child's troubles ought to be over. Monitor the diet of younger kids carefully, and teach older children to find out exactly what they are going to eat by reading labels or asking questions. *Do not slip up!* If you and they exercise care, the kids should be out of harm's way. There are, however, two possible complica-

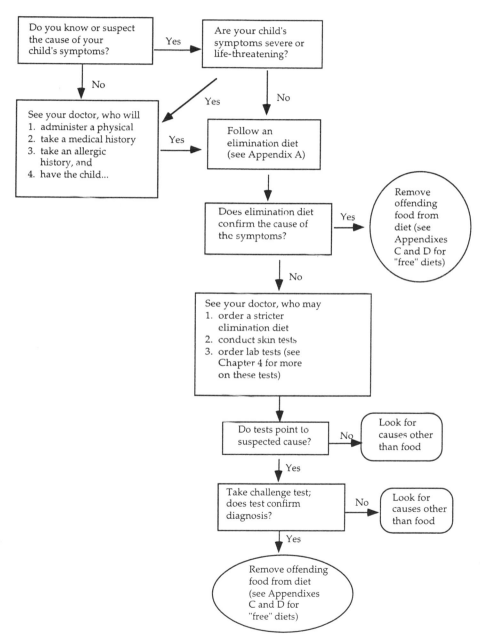

Fig. 5. Steps in identification of food hypersensitivity or allergy.

tions: The offending food or substance may occur in unexpected places. (Milk or milk protein turns up in everything from bologna to zabaglione; tartrazine is apparently ritually cast into nearly everything processed or prepared.) Of special interest is the fact that some products that are milk-free are found to be cross-contaminated in the process of manufacture! Follow the "free" diets in Appendixes C and D to sidestep these problems. The offender may come from a big family. Cross-sensitivity happens frequently in food intolerances, so that if mustard greens make your child's stomach ache, for instance, all of the members of the mustard family—turnip, radish, horseradish, watercress, cabbage, Chinese cabbage, broccoli, and the many other members of this clan—may also do so. Appendix B gives families of foods that cross-react.

Avoidance is the safest and most effective tactic to follow in controlling food intolerance symptoms. If complete avoidance is not possible (because the list of irritants is long and diffuse) and if the sensitivity is truly immunological or allergic, then suppressing symptoms through medication is sometimes a workable alternative. *This control step should be taken only under medical supervision.*

Special Hints

As we noted in the preceding section, when you do isolate the source of the reaction, your child's problems are over—almost. Along the way, however, there are a few things to know and to be careful about.

A special problem shows up in young children. As we pointed out above, infants and very young children often absorb small quantities of undigested food. As children grow older, however, their gastrointestinal tracts mature, food comes to be digested completely and absorption of small quantities of undigested food no longer occurs. With this maturation of the intestine and proper food digestion, the symptoms of food allergy generally disappear. However, if these children go on to develop pollen sensitivity (hay fever) their food allergies may return.

Skin tests or oral challenges should not be done if the child's food intolerance is severe or life-threatening. Skin tests (scratch or prick) for food hypersensitivity are crude, cover only a minute fraction of the possibilities, are potentially dangerous, and are useful mainly in their ability to identify lack of sensitivity to a substance. A course of skin tests will likely eliminate some suspects, turn up a few false leads (false positive reactions) and, perhaps, the real culprit.

Challenge tests are the key to definitive identification of specific causes of food hypersensitivity (*see* Chapter 4 for more on challenge tests).

11

Asthma (Wheezing and Shortness of Breath)

There are few, if any, ailments which have terrified children and their families more and more often than wheezing and asthma.[*]

Asthma accounts for more absences from school than any other chronic illness and is a leading cause of visits to the doctor's office. It is a serious disease—the death rate among hospitalized asthmatic children is under 1%, but rises to 24% in adults.

More than two-thirds of asthmatics have a family member—brother, sister, or parent—who has or has had asthma, but the hereditary basis for the complaint is complex and not completely understood. Some children from families riddled with the complaint never show the disease; others from seemingly clear backgrounds inexplicably turn up with it.

Incidence

Asthma (which originally meant "shortness of breath") is among the most common of ailments—up to 5% of Americans, 10 million people suffer from it. Recent studies indicate that one in nine Californians has the disease.

In childhood, it is one-third more common and more severe in males, but after puberty, the sex distribution is about even. It is more often found in urban, industrialized settings, in colder climates, and among the urban disadvantaged, especially African-Americans.

---

[*]For a detailed discussion of asthma, its symptoms, causes, and treatment, *see* Gershwin, M. E. and Klingelhofer, E. L. *Asthma: Stop Suffering, Start Living,* 2nd ed. Addison-Wesley Publishing, Reading, MA, 1992.

Usual Age of Onset

Asthma may turn up at any age, although the first episode is likely to occur between the second and fifth years. In a few children, wheezing and shortness of breath are evident right from birth.

Symptoms

Asthma is a collection of respiratory symptoms, the most prominent of which are shortness of breath, wheezing, coughing, and increased production of mucus.

The shortness of breath (which can be sudden in onset) and wheezing are produced by "twitchiness" of the respiratory airways.

As air is inhaled through either the nose or the mouth, it flows through a series of airways. These airways—tubes, really—begin in the throat and descend all the way down to the base of the lungs. At the level of the throat and upper chest, they are fairly large. The uppermost and largest is called the trachea. About one-third of the way down into the chest, the trachea branches into two somewhat smaller airways known as main stem bronchi. Each of these main stem bronchi supplies air to one of the lungs.

As the bronchi extend deeper and deeper into the chest, the air tubes proliferate and become smaller and smaller. The result is a complex maze of small tubes—airways—which resemble the root structure of a tree. Surrounding these airways is a layer of smooth muscle. This muscle maintains the size and shape of the airways. In asthmatics, the muscle is "spastic" or "twitchy"—likely to go into a spasm when stimulated by any of a number of factors. When the smooth muscle sheath does go into spasm, it chokes or constricts the airways thus making less room for the air to move in and out of the lung. It is this restriction of air flow that produces the high-pitched wheezing and the struggle to breathe that are characteristic of asthma.

In addition to the layer of spastic muscle tissue around the airways, mucus producing cells called goblet cells are important contributors to asthma. Everybody, whether normal or asthmatic, has these mucus-producing cells. Mucus is important because it carries the enzymes and chemicals that help the lungs to fight infection. In asthmatics, however, there is an increase in the number of mucus cells, with the number increasing with the severity of asthma. These cells produce an excess of mucus, which clogs airways and obstructs the flow of air. This is especially true in the small airways at the bottom of the lungs.

Causes

Asthma has many different causes or triggers, both allergic and non-allergic. In children, the most prominent ones are respiratory infections, airborne allergens, food additives, vigorous exercise, and exposure to cold, dry air. Asthma symptoms are also associated with cyctic fibrosis and gastroesophageal reflux (GER), rare but grave conditions in infants and children.

When to See the Doctor

Regardless of its severity, the very first wheezing episode should signal you to call your doctor even if the episode is mild and transient. At that appointment, the doctor will take a medical history and carry out a physical examination, order a chest X-ray, and, if necessary, give allergy skin tests.

A medical history and a complete physical examination are vital to the management of asthma. The physical should include measures of height, weight, blood pressure, pulse, and assessment of any other possible asthma-contributing factors. The chest should be very carefully listened to by the doctor to determine if there might be an anatomic basis for obstruction. A tumor or a foreign body in the airway also causes a decrease in airflow and a wheeze. (Asthma is a symmetric disease affecting both sides of the chest; an obstruction is likely to affect only one side—perhaps only a section of one lung on one side. Careful listening can pick up this difference.)

At this early stage, your child should have a chest X-ray. It is usually not necessary to repeat chest X-rays thereafter, but an initial picture will help identify any potential anatomic problems and will be useful for later reference. Following the physical examination, the physician and you must decide whether allergy skin tests are needed.

Skin Testing

Skin tests entail making a series of minor scratches or pricks on the skin and introducing different allergen extracts into these wounds; the substances to which one is allergic will quickly develop a raised, white patch with a surrounding redness of the skin.

Allergy skin tests that help to determine what is causing the wheezing and shortness of breath are among the most abused of all procedures in medicine. Many physicians, believing they are more accurate than they really are, carry out wholesale testing with allergic antigens. These antigens are often very crude; sometimes the test procedures irritate the skin and produce false-positive results, that is, a reaction owing not to an antibody or allergy but rather to a simple irritation that has nothing to do with allergy.

There are several factors that determine whether an asthmatic child should have skin testing. *Children under age 4 should be skin tested only under exceptional conditions.* If allergy skin tests are to be performed, which ones are administered should be determined by where you live and how the disease manifests itself. Allergy skin tests can be divided into several categories. The most common are those using pollens, the tests for which are made from extracts of trees, weeds, and grasses. The child should be skin tested with pollens found in the locale—a Californian should not be tested with midwestern weeds. Then, there are the mold antigens. Molds are found almost everywhere, and many asthmatics are allergic to them. Third, there are the environmental agents that test reactions to things found in the home, especially house dust and animal danders. Finally, there are extracts that purport to detect sensitivity to certain foods. These last tests should rarely be used; they are very crude and unlikely to yield clinically important information. If food allergy is suspected, then the physician should carry out a special challenge test of the sort described in Chapter 4.

Occasionally, a bronchial challenge is carried out, usually in a hospital setting. If your youngster's symptoms are confusing or contradictory, he or she may be asked to inhale a vapor containing an allergen (often a pollen); sometimes the vapor will contain a chemical called methacholine. The reason for this test is to find out what causes the wheezing and to determine if the child really has asthma. Over 90% of asthmatics will show asthmatic symptoms when methacholine is inhaled; generally fewer than 10% of those who do not have asthma will have a positive reaction. If the results of the metacholine test are positive, you can be fairly sure that your child does in fact have asthma even though you and the doctor may still not know what is causing it.

Some circumstances call for an asthmatic child to have a four-way CT scan of the sinuses. It has been discovered that untreated and undiagnosed sinusitis can make asthma more difficult to treat. A four-way CT scan is cheaper and subjects the child to considerably less radiation than old fashioned X-rays.

Treatment of Asthma

Effective treatment of asthma entails following five rather complicated steps. Not all are applicable to everyone. The steps are:

1. Identification of causal agents.
2. Avoidance of causal agents.
3. Control of appearance of symptoms through medication and other strategies.
4. Treatment of symptoms.
5. Prevention and/or reduction of symptoms through allergy shots.

Identify the Causal Agent or Agents

There are a large number of factors that can precipitate asthma attacks. The most important ones are:

Colds or upper respiratory infections;
Exposure to allergens;
Vigorous exercise;

Emotional responses including hyperventilation;
Certain drugs, especially aspirin;
Air pollutants including tobacco smoke, ozone, and sulfur dioxide;
Preservatives in food, especially metabisulfite.

Some brief comments about the causal agents may help you in your search for the one—or ones—that are responsible for your child's asthma.

Colds or upper respiratory infections are the most common forerunners of asthmatic attacks in children. The cold symptoms—sneezing, sniffling, coughing, stuffy nose, sore throat, possibly a slight fever—usually appear before asthma takes hold. Then the congestion will become worse, the chest will feel constricted, and shortness of breath, deeper coughing, and wheezing will show up. These asthmatic symptoms may persist well after the main infection is largely gone.

Up to half or all asthmatic children show allergies to pollens, house dust, animals, foods, or molds, but these allergies are not necessarily the major cause of their asthmatic reactions. Often, they are however, if the child has a high level of IgE antibodies.

Foods draw much unwarranted suspicion as causes of asthma. The idea that your child's asthma can be provoked by some mysterious, insidious allergy to foods is largely unfounded. Foods seldom cause asthma. Food additives can and do though, particularly tartrazine, which is found in food dye color #5 (FDC#5), a yellow dye used in potato chips, tacos, and other yellow candy and processed foods. The incidence of tartrazine-induced asthma is much less than once believed, but is still a factor in some patients. Common foods containing tartrazine are listed in Appendix D-4.

Exercise is frequently implicated in bronchospasm. Interestingly, the form of exercise has much to do with it. Swimming is relatively harmless and unlikely to provoke airway collapse in asthmatics, but running or jogging often will. Whether or not exercise will cause your child to wheeze also depends on the temperature and humidity of the air breathed—the more moist and the warmer the air, the less the likelihood of wheezing. Wherever possible, we encourage all children with asthma to become regular swimmers.

Emotional responses—anger and fear in particular—have long been blamed for causing asthma. Although an emotional state like the anger or resentment that accompanies or follows conflict between parent and child does not induce asthma, it can cause rapid, shallow breathing or hyperventilation. This hyperventilation in children with twitchy airways brings on bronchospasm and wheezing. There are probably other ways in which emotional reactions induce bronchospasm—recent evidence hints at a relationship between certain personality traits and asthma. However, the underlying ways—the mechanisms—by which traits generate symptoms—if, in fact they do—are still unknown.

Many drugs, particularly those classified as nonsteroidal anti-inflammatory drugs (aspirin and its relatives) can induce violent asthmatic reactions. If your child has asthma, steer clear of aspirin and all other nonsteroidal drugs.

Patty's asthma always gets worse with her period. She knows to avoid aspirin, but takes Advil to ease her pain and discomfort. Advil is a drug called ibuprofen, which is an aspirin imitator. Patty was never told that there are hundreds of drugs that contain aspirin and aspirin look-alikes. These drugs are called nonsteroidal anti-inflammatory agents. Tylenol (acetaminophen) is not an aspirin look-alike and is generally safe. (A list of some of these products is in Table 8.)

Air pollution, especially from sulfur dioxide, ozone, and the particulate pollutants resulting from the combustion of fossil fuels cause twitchy airways to become worse. In addition to atmospheric pollutants, tobacco smoke—first-hand or second-hand—is an important triggering agent for asthma and should be studiously avoided.

Avoid Asthma's Causal Agents

Once you identify the agents responsible for your child's asthma, the next step is to design effective ways of avoiding contact with them.

Avoiding exposure to colds and respiratory infections is fairly difficult. Chapter 5 spells out the steps you and your child can take to cut the risk of colds.

If vigorous exercise pushes your child into an asthmatic attack, he or she has three options: exercise anyway and suffer the consequences, substitute another activity, or take medication beforehand. For the first two alternatives, nothing more needs to be said. If the child wants to do demanding sports or activities that provoke asthmatic reactions, Jim's experience may be instructive.

Jim has had asthma all of his 15 years. He is particularly troubled by wheezing during physical exercise in school and is unable to keep up with the other boys on account of it. His doctor says that he has exercise-induced asthma and has recommended that he take theophylline, an older but still widely used form of treatment. Jim cannot tolerate theophylline, which gives him an upset stomach and nausea, and he would much rather stay out of physical education than take the medication. Jim's parents consulted another physician who recommended that he use an albuterol inhaler prior to exercise. Although school rules forbid students to carry handheld nebulizers in their pockets, they do make it available in the school nurse's office, so Jim goes there immediately before his gym class. Since he started doing this, he has improved greatly in stamina and, to his immense satisfaction, his athletic skills have picked up, too.

Asthma is a rich source of emotional reactions.

- Asthmatics and their parents experience frustration, fear, panic, and guilt over the attacks.

- Children having moderate to severe attacks spend a lot of time wondering if they are going to die this time.
- Parents understandably become oversolicitous and overprotective of their asthmatic children, keeping them from participating in and enjoying ordinary activities, from developing normally, and in doing this, forging an undesirably close dependency which may be difficult to break in later life.
- Parents and nonasthmatic brothers and sisters quite often resent the attention, the care, and the expenditures that the asthmatic requires.
- Asthmatics may use their condition to have their way in the family or elsewhere.

If you establish that asthma in your child has an emotional base—if attacks have more than a coincidental relationship to other events that cause conflict, stress, anger, or frustration—teaching the child how to breathe when having an emotional reaction will help. The youngster should, at times of stress or tension, be taught to:

1. Sit down in a quiet place. Turning the chair so that the child has nothing but the wall to look at is useful.
2. Take slow, deliberate, deep breaths, inhaling through the mouth and exhaling slowly through the nose.
3. Continue this for a short period of time—usually no more than 5 minutes should be enough to restore the youngster's ordinary breathing rhythm and reverse the bronchospasms.

Billy used to wheeze during the cowboy movies as a youngster. His mom used to tease him that it was from the dust being kicked up by the galloping horses on the silver screen. Actually Billy was fully involved in the action, overexcited, and hyperventilating as a result.

To avoid some of the major difficulties growing out of emotional responses, keep the communication lines open. Discuss problems frankly and directly as they come up. Do not let them fester. Also, do not treat your asthmatic children as invalids. If you do, they may start believing you.

Drugs

Any time your child sees a doctor or gets a prescription, remind the physician without fail, that the youngster is asthmatic.

By following four simple rules, you can help your child avoid drug-induced asthma.

1. Monitor the child's reactions carefully after the use of any drug.
2. NEVER self-administer aspirin or any other nonsteroidal anti-inflammatory drugs or medications.

3. NEVER administer any drug without first letting your doctor know about it and consulting him or the *Physician's Desk Reference* (which is available in public libraries or the doctor's office) for possible side effects—especially asthmatic ones.
4. ALWAYS use a peak flow meter and record the readings in a diary.

The most common and serious of the *air pollutants is tobacco smoke. Asthmatic children should not smoke tobacco, they should avoid the tobacco smoke of others, and members of their household must not smoke.*

High concentrations of ozone and sulfur dioxide—air pollution—are the results of a conspiracy of climatic conditions and automobile emissions, which cause asthmatics considerable distress. Here is what to do if you and your child wind up in a smog-filled city.

Most cities with significant smog problems forecast air quality, and the forecast for the Pollution Standards Index (PSI) will appear in the morning newspaper. If the index is to be "high" or "alert" (ordinarily a value of 100 or more), then it will be especially dangerous for your asthmatic child, because the pollutant indexes apply to normal people; people with respiratory disease start showing symptoms when the index is "moderate"—in the 70 range. When that happens or is about to happen, keep your child indoors. Keep the windows closed. Have the youngster curl up with a good book or in front of the television set. Do not let the child play out-of-doors until the air quality improves. If the youngster must go out, then have him or her wear a disposable mask. Effective paper masks, much like those worn by surgeons or carpenters, are available at your drug store. The mask will not affect the level of sulfur dioxide or other gas, but will filter out some particulate matter. While outside in these conditions, asthmatic children should not exercise or otherwise exert themselves. They should walk at a moderate pace and avoid other obvious triggering factors in the environment, like automobile emissions and tobacco smoke.

Control Symptoms Through Clearance of Mucus, Breathing Exercises, and Medication

Very often asthmatic symptoms—wheezing, shortness of breath, coughing—can be kept from developing or can be controlled, if they appear, by using a combination of measures. These control measures include clearing the mucus, improving the airways through breathing exercises, and using medicine intelligently. The sections that follow tell you how you can put these measures into practice.

Getting Rid of Mucus: During an asthma attack, the goblet cells that line the airways, drastically increase their production of mucus. When this sticky, tenacious material lodges in the airways it makes breathing even more difficult for your asthmatic child. Sometimes it gets so bad that asthmatics literally drown in their own phlegm.

There is nothing you can do to affect the production of mucus, but there are simple and effective steps you can take to keep it thin and easy to move. To keep mucus from getting dangerously thick and clingy, your child must drink at least two full glasses of water four times per day. Warm water is best for this purpose—stay away from juices, sodas, milk, or other beverages that carry the possibility of allergic complications and do not get absorbed by the body any faster. Spicy foods have also been found to loosen mucus. Adding 10 to 20 drops of Tabasco sauce to a glass of 8 ounces of water would be an appropriate dose for adolescent asthmatics. Getting the mucus out is a bit more difficult. However, it can be done readily enough provided you devote time to it and help your child in the process. What you will be doing, in fact, is getting the phlegm *down* and out, because you will have the child take a series of positions where the chest and torso will be higher than the head, and the mucus, aided by your gentle tapping, will be dislodged and ooze out of the airways. To do this, you will need a stiff, wedge-shaped bolster a couple of feet square and at least 4 to 6 inches higher at one end.

You will have the child lie on the bolster, belt line at the high end, head on the floor at the low end, back down, then left side down, and then right side down, then front down (Illustration 1).

In each position, tap the uppermost part of the child's chest gently with your fingers. This will loosen the clinging mucus and speed its outward flow. A handheld vibrator will also work (Illustration 2). For best results have the child stay in each position from 3 to 5 minutes. You will want to do the mucus clearing twice a day. Sleep will also be improved if you schedule one session just before the child goes to bed.

Improving Breathing: You can greatly reduce the severity of asthmatic attacks if you teach your child to breathe properly.

There are three different kinds of exercises that will improve your child's breathing. The first kind teaches how to involve the diaphragm in the process of breathing—something that most people do not do.

1. Have the child locate the diaphragm (which is a large, powerful muscle) by putting his hands on the stomach between navel and rib cage (Illustration 3A).
2. Keeping hands on the diaphragm, have the child take a deep breath. If the diaphragm is being used, the hands will be pushed forward. Then exhale; the hands should now move inward.
3. Once you get the child to the point where he or she can move the diaphragm, have him or her practice diaphragmatic breathing four

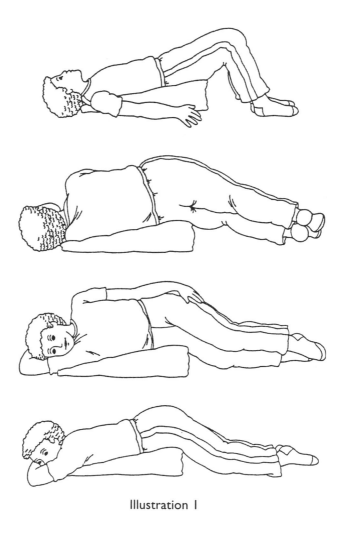

Illustration I

times a day for 3 or 4 minutes each time. Keep the hands on the diaphragm always; do the breathing exercise standing for 1 minute, sitting for 1 minute, and reclining on the back for 1 minute (Illustration 3).

4. When, after a week or so, diaphragmatic breathing becomes automatic, add this exercise. With the child lying on the back, place a weight—3 to 5 pounds of books are about right—on the diaphragm. Have the child breathe in deeply, using the diaphragm, and then exhale slowly. Repeat this exercise 10 times, twice daily. This will strengthen the diaphragm (Illustration 4).

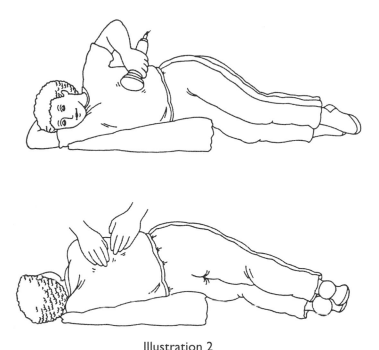

Illustration 2

The second kind of breathing exercise helps expand the child's rib cage and get unused lung cells into action.

1. Have the child lock fingers behind the neck and press the elbows back while inhaling. Hold the breath a few seconds, and then exhale while bringing the elbows together in front. (This exercise can be done sitting, standing, or lying down.) Repeat 10 times, twice a day (Illustration 5).
2. Have the child sit upright. Raise the arms high while inhaling, then slowly bend forward and exhale slowly. The hands should touch the floor. Repeat 10 times, twice a day (Illustration 6).
3. Sit the child upright. Put one hand flat on the stomach and extend the other arm out horizontally and away from the body while inhaling deeply. Exhale slowly while bringing the hand of the extended arm to the opposite shoulder. Repeat, alternating positions of hands, 10 times, twice daily (Illustration 7).

As you know, the bronchial tubes have walls of smooth muscle, and it is this muscle that contracts and causes wheezing and shortness of breath. Your child's bronchial walls can be strengthened and made more resistant to spasm through the following exercise. Have the child clench the fingers of

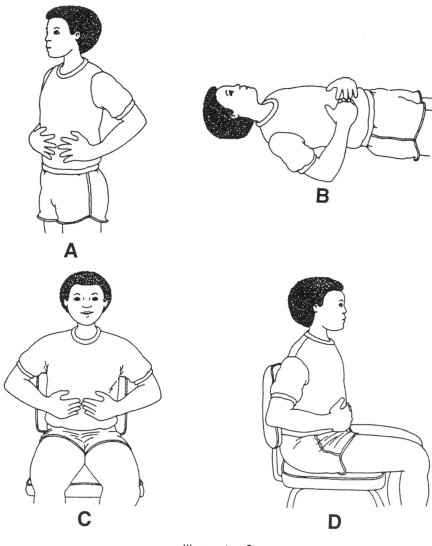

A

B

C

D

Illustration 3

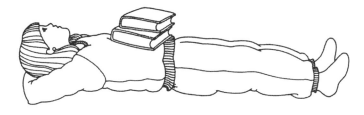

Illustration 4

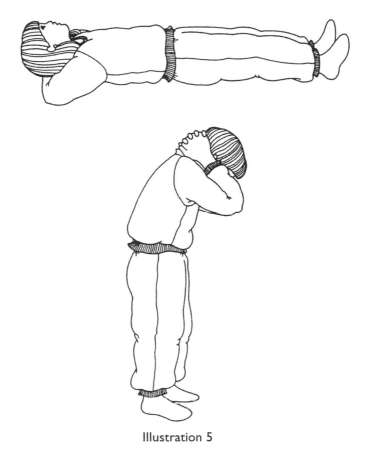

Illustration 5

one hand in order to make a closed cylinder (the kind of arrangement you make when the hands are cold and you blow on them to warm them.) See that the cylinder is as tight as possible. Have the child blow into it, remove it from mouth, inhale, and blow again with increasing force. Do this for a minute or two, three times daily (Illustration 8).

These breathing exercises, if done faithfully, will increase your child's lung capacity, muscle tone, and resistance to asthmatic bronchospasm.

Controlling or Treating Asthmatic Symptoms with Medication or Drugs

There are several medications available that keep asthma symptoms from appearing or relieve them when they are present. These medications are beta-agonists, theophyllines, cromolyn, leukotriene inhibitors, and corticosteroids (cortisone). Except for a few over-the-counter beta-agonists, these are all prescription drugs and must be ordered by your doctor. They are appropriate for use if your

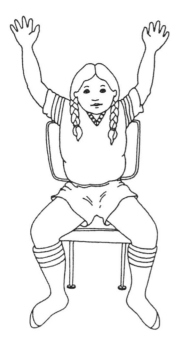 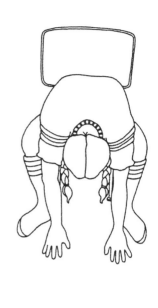

Illustration 6

child is moderately to severely asthmatic. The paragraphs below and Table 10 tell how the drugs act, what forms they take, the ages for which they are appropriate, their advantages, and their disadvantages.

Beta-agonists are the major class of medications for asthma. These drugs can be taken orally, but are most commonly and effectively administered by operating a metered, handheld, aerosol canister. They provide rapid relief of asthmatic wheezing and shortness of breath. Activating the canister releases a puff of drug-saturated aerosol, which is carried directly to the twitchy smooth muscle in the airways. This direct action quells the symptoms much more rapidly than the theophyllines do. Since they work almost instantaneously, they are extremely satisfying to use.

There are over-the-counter aerosols available. Primatene Mist and Bronkaid, the two most heavily advertised ones, are effective for the treatment of occasional very mild symptoms and have sometimes helped children who suffer from this very mild asthma. However, they are not as effective as new prescription drugs and are more toxic.

Beta-agonists are the first line of treatment for asthma, because they have fewer side effects, they are more convenient, and they act more rapidly. The effectiveness of aerosols depends very much on knowing how to use them effectively. *DO NOT OVERUSE THEM* (2 inhalations every 4 hours and not more than 12 puffs per day).

To use a metered aerosol effectively, teach your child to follow these steps:

1. Shake inhaler.
2. Begin inhalation and, at the same time, place aerosol just in front of the mouth at a distance of 1 to 2 inches, and release a properly aimed puff of aerosol (aerosol should go straight to the large airways; it should not impact at the back of the throat).*
3. Inhale at a moderate rate with open mouth.
4. Hold breath for 5 seconds.
5. Exhale.

For more severe asthmatics and for very young children, we use solutions of beta-agonists given by nebulization (*see below*).

Theophyllines are related to caffeine and work by relaxing bronchial smooth muscle, thus opening up the airways and making breathing easier. The amount of theophylline to take depends on body size and has to be determined carefully. Even then there are sometimes significant differences in reactions between like-sized individuals, so physicians, when prescribing theophylline, ought to order a blood test that measures how much theophylline is in the blood several days after starting to take it.

When taken regularly (and with careful initial monitoring of the blood to detect potentially dangerous side effects), theophylline keeps wheezing from developing and permits asthmatics to lead a much more comfortable and normal life.

Theophyllines come in four forms:

1. A liquid;
2. A chewable tablet;
3. A pill; and
4. A capsule containing time-release beads.

The liquid form, such as slophylline, is very disagreeable to taste—a problem found in all the theophylline elixirs and suspensions. They are definitely

---

*To direct the spray efficiently, "spacers" are often useful. A cheap, effective spacing device is the cardboard cylinder found within a roll of toilet paper. With seals between the mouth and the metered aerosol, it works quite well. A small plastic container made into a simple cylinder has also been shown to be an effective delivery system. Many commercial spacers are available—ask your pharmacist for help in choosing one.

These spacers simply hold the aerosol in suspension for several seconds. The child who is unable to inhale the aerosol successfully thus has more than one inspiration to get the medication to the lungs.

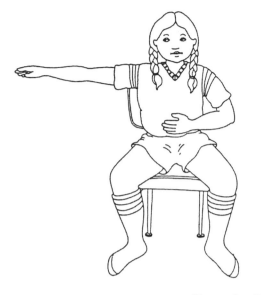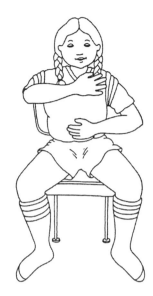

Illustration 7

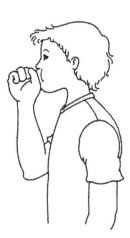

Illustration 8

not recommended.

The chewable tablets are only rarely better tasting than the liquid versions and are also *not* recommended.

The tablets, such as Theodur and Respid, are preferable for children who can swallow pills.

The time-release capsules, when swallowed, are as effective as the tablets and some of them, Slo-Bid, for example, can be opened and the beads spread over applesauce or yogurt, making it very easy for young children to swallow them. There is even a special preparation of theophylline, called Theodur-sprinkle, that is made just for this purpose. When giving theophylline to young children, we recommend the bead or sprinkle, although your doctor must still check the child's blood to verify the levels of drug. Checking blood levels of theophylline is important for all patients and is imperative for young children, since often the beads or sprinkles do not get absorbed. Theophyllines, regardless of their form, because of their toxicity are rarely the first line of treatment in the management of asthma.

Cromolyn sodium a chemical originally isolated from an Egyptian weed, comes in two forms: as a metered aerosol, or as a liquid for nebulization. The metered dose of cromolyn (Intal) is administered in the same way as the beta-agonists. The liquid for nebulization is delivered as noted below. Cromolyn, and its newer cousin, Tilade, are not first-line drugs in asthma but they can be very helpful second-line or third-line defenses.

Cromolyn should be given a fair and serious trial by the young child who is not responding to other therapy. It is often not totally effective when given alone to control moderate to severe asthma. Thus, it works best when teamed with other drugs, such as beta-agonists or inhaled steroids. These comments aside, Intal and Tilade have almost no toxicity.

Leukotriene inhibitors. Asthma is best viewed as a syndrome of chronic inflammation. To help combat the inflammation, newer drugs are being developed. These drugs are designed to inhibit the formation of leukotrienes, because leukotrienes have been shown to make asthma worse. Two products have recently been approved by the FDA. The first of these is Accolate® (Zafirlukast) for usage in adults and teenagers. It is prescribed as a pill to be taken twice a day, 1 hour before or 2 hours after meals. It works best in mild and moderate asthma. The second drug is Zyflo® (Zileuton). It is also for usage only in teenagers and adults. Its usual dosage is 1 tablet 4 times a day with or without food. Some patients experience some mild liver problems with Zyflo® and it is recommended that liver function tests be followed. For both drugs, drug interactions are possible, and your doctor should be aware of every other drug being taken. Zyflo® works best in moderate to severe asthma. However, both of these agents offer a significant and new class of agents that may help patients with asthma. We should also note that these new drugs work by prevention and must be taken on a regular basis to be effective. They are not indicated for the treatment of acute asthma. The safety and effectiveness of these drugs in young children have not been established.

Steroids, drugs in the cortisone family, are useful in two ways. Taken orally or intravenously, they are helpful for children with very severe asthma—children who are hospitalized. Delivered in this form, steroids can be life-saving, but they carry significant negative side effects.

Steroids are also available in topical as opposed to systemic forms, in aerosols much like beta-agonists. When properly taken, they act only on the lungs and do not carry the negative side effects associated with the other forms. These aerosol steroids can be quite effective in improving breathing. Although they do not deliver the amount of cortisone required for severe (but unhospitalized) asthmatics, they are extremely helpful in subacute cases. These agents include Beclovent, Vanceril, Aerobid, Azmacort, and Flovent. Flovent, the newest of the lot, has only recently been approved and is the only such drug available in three different concentrations. It easily appears to be the best of these topical steroids, and some patients do well when using Flovent as their only drug. Another topical steroid, Aero-Bid, is unpleasant to take because it has a bad taste and often induces nausea; it is therefore *not* recommended even when packaged with a mint flavor.

Nebulizers: For very young children and for children who have very severe asthma, a more effective and immediate treatment is often needed. About 15 years ago, it was realized that a simple air compressor, when used to blow air through a solution of medicine, would create a fine aerosol of medicine—a nebula—which could be rapidly inhaled into the lung. The development of home nebulization equipment has been one of the most important advances in the management of asthma. The most popular nebulizers are made by DeVilbiss Inc., P. O. Box 35, Somerset, PA 15501. Some units will operate off rechargeable batteries, wall current, or the cigarette lighter in your car. These units cost from $200 to $400 and, when prescribed by your doctor, are paid for by most insurance companies. Patients who cannot afford them can often get them for free from local respiratory societies or rent them at a nominal cost.

> Chrissy, now 12, has had asthma nearly all of her life. For her first several years, she had to have shots of adrenaline up to 30 times a year to control her symptoms. At age 6, her doctor prescribed a Pulmo-Aid. Since that time, Chrissy has not required a single injection. She takes her Albuterol by nebulization, and now plays softball and plays flute in the school band.

If your child is moderately to severely asthmatic, you should discuss the possibility and appropriateness of a nebulizer with your physician.

How to Monitor Your Asthma

Consistent and informed use of a peak flow meter is essential to the management of asthmatic symptoms. By using it daily to record the peak expiratory flow rate (PEFR), the maximum speed with which air can be exhaled, the status of the lungs can be monitored, and decreases from the typical or normal rate can signal the need for corrective action. There are several different makes of meters available; they range in cost from $20 to $30, and all come with instructions for use and care of the meter, performance norms by age, size, and gender, and materials for recording performance.

Proper use of a flow meter entails:

1. Defining a normal or baseline PEFR, preferably in consultation with the physician.
2. Using the meter at least twice daily, morning and evening. Taking three measures at each session and recording the highest of them. (Faithful observance of this step is crucial.)
3. Comparing the reading with the norm; if the session's reading is 80% or more of the norm, OK.
4. If the reading is less than 80% of normal, take whatever precautionary steps may be indicated, based on past experience and advice from your physician. (Depending on the amount of fall-off, this may be a signal to wait and see, to start medication, to increase medication, or to call the doctor.)

Conscientious use of a peak flow meter will give a dependable day-by-day view of respiratory health and is probably the single best preventive step that asthmatics can take—and it does not hurt to remember that, when prescribed by your doctor, your insurance company will almost certainly pick up the tab for it.

Special Hints or Warnings

It will help parents to note and remember the following points:

1. The belief that asthma is psychologically-caused is a myth. If your child has asthma it is because of his genes; nothing is the matter with his emotional life although there may be, in time, if you act as if you believed the old misconception that asthma springs from psychological roots.
2. The most difficult aspect of asthma for parents is the acute concern, sometimes verging on dread, they experience when they see their child fighting for breath in the grip of a moderate attack.

Note carefully:

- The breathlessness usually seems more severe than it is. Do not panic.
- *Do not* advise the child to breathe deeply. This can actually make the symptoms worse. Let the child find his or her own respiratory rhythm.
- *Do not* encourage the child to cough. This can force mucus into the airways, further compromising the breathing.
- *Do not* administer any drugs other than the ones prescribed by

your physician. In particular, *never* give an asthmatic child seda-
tives, tranquilizers, or aspirin in any form (helping a child go to
sleep can be extremely dangerous).

- Administer all medications exactly as prescribed in the amount and
according to the schedule your doctor orders. (If you are not clear
about what to do, clarify your responsibilities completely before
leaving the doctor's office; do not undermedicate or overmedicate.)
- If the youngster's condition gets to the point where you cannot
help and seems to be worsening, do not hesitate to call the doctor
or go to the emergency room. The belief that asthmatics wheeze
their way into old age is false; they do *if,* they get proper and
timely care.
- Resist the temptation to seek treatment from chiropractors,
herbalists, naturopaths, homeopaths, "organic," "psychic," or
other unconventional "healers." They have nothing to offer
that will effectively relieve the smooth muscle spasms that
trigger asthma.

3. Be wary about putting your child through a course of allergy shots
for the prevention of asthma. In no case should a young child have
them; an older child might be helped by shots *if* it is definitely known
that the asthma is a reaction to an allergen, *if* there is an effective
antigen available, *if* strict and carefully observed avoidance tactics
have not worked, and *if* medications have proved ineffectual.

4. If your child is severely and chronically afflicted with asthma, consider
getting a home air compressor (Pulmo-aide), which is an especially
effective way of delivering beta-agonists or cromolyn (*see above*).

5. Take heart from the knowledge that asthma, because of the physiology that underlies the disease, improves as children grow older.
Although they do not get rid of the disease (the tendency for the
airway smooth muscle to become spastic is still there), the airways
enlarge, the symptoms decline in severity, and eventually fade
away to the point where they are no longer evident to you or the
child. Being patient, knowledgeable, and doing the right things
when they need doing will speed this process along.

6. You can probably reduce the frequency, severity, and costs of your
child's asthma attacks materially by getting involved in a childhood Asthma Self-Management Program. There are half a dozen
or so of these programs around, and they are increasingly being
made available through HMOs, hospitals, your local American
Lung Association branch, or the Asthma and Allergy Foundation
of America. These programs offer instruction, useful strategies,

Table 9
Asthma Medications for Children

Medication	Example	Advantages	Disadvantages
Theophyllines	Respid Slo-Bid Theodur Theodur- 　Sprinkle	An effective drug 　for mild and 　moderate asthma	Slow to act; strong stimulant affecting 　activity level and behavior; can cause 　sleep disorders; stomach upset; increase 　in urine output; sometimes toxic, 　especially when upper respiratory 　infections are present
Beta-Agonists	Alupent Albuterol	Works quickly; 　convenient to 　carry; can be 　called into use as 　soon as needed	Difficult to take effectively (see text); can 　cause heartbeat irregularities, chest 　pain, muscle tremors, nausea, vomiting, 　dizziness, weakness, sweating. 　Available as solution for nebulization
	Brethaire	Works quickly	Tolerance can develop. Not recommended
	Bitoterol	Longer duration of 　action—6 to 　8 hours	Takes 1/2 hour to work; not recommended
	Salmeterol	Convenient twice 　a day dosing	Can be toxic if overused; not studied in 　young children
Cromolyn 　(Intal)	Powder	Very effective for 　allergy and 　exercise-induced 　asthma; few 　side effects	Can cause coughing and aggravate 　breathing difficulties
	Inhaler	Easier to use than 　powder	Sometimes not as effective as powder
	Nebulized 　solution	Dramatically improves 　delivery in young 　children	Requires a nebulizer
Tilade	Inhaler	Effective in prevention	Not as effective as inhaled steroids
Leukotriene 　inhibitor	Accolate	Taken orally; little 　toxicity	Only effective in mild or moderate 　asthma
	Zyflo®	Good for moderate 　to severe asthma	Liver function tests should be monitored
Steroids	Prednisone	Very good for severe 　asthma	Carries major and dangerous side effects
	Beclomethasone Azmacort	Acts on lungs only; 　side effects 　minimal when 　taken properly	Not effective for acutely ill children; 　allergy to vehicle may develop; can 　trigger coughing and wheezing in 　some children
	Aerobid	None	Disagreeable taste, not recommended
	Flo-Vent	Comes in three doses	Not effective for acutely ill children
Anticholinergic	Atrovent	Low toxicity; may 　reduce cough	Not a first-line drug for asthma; best for 　chronic bronchitis of adults
	Combi-Vent	A combination of 　Atrovent and 　Albuteral	Can be useful for older children

and/or practice in a variety of skills or procedures that, when followed faithfully, help to prevent or control asthma attacks. To be put in touch with these programs in your area, contact your American Lung Association branch, the allergy department of your HMO, or your child's physician.

7. If you need help with a problem or an answer to a question about asthma, the National Asthma Center in Denver, Colorado has a toll-free number you can call. The number is 800-222-LUNG.

12

Hay Fever (Allergic Rhinitis and Chronic Runny Nose)

Children, from birth on, are subject to runny noses. The main reasons are upper respiratory infections—colds and allergies—although a few youngsters do have chronic runny noses for no discernible reason.

When the runny nose is the result of an allergy, the condition is called allergic rhinitis. Most allergic rhinitis is a reaction to plant pollens and is popularly known as hay fever. However, a large number of airborne substances, including house dust, mold, chemicals, and dander from animals, provoke symptoms identical to those of hay fever. This condition is simply called perennial or year-long allergic rhinitis. From a medical standpoint, the terms hay fever and allergic rhinitis are synonyms.

Incidence

Allergic rhinitis is the most common allergy; over 20 million Americans have it. The seasonal form (hay fever) is twice as prevalent as the perennial variety (allergic reactions to house dust, mold, and so on). In the first 10 years of life, boys are more likely to have allergic rhinitis than girls. If either parent has allergic rhinitis, their children are three to five times more likely to have allergic rhinitis than they would be if the parents were free of the disease.

Usual Age of Onset

Allergic rhinitis develops after a period of sensitization has taken place; hay fever, with its intermittent seasonal exposure to pollens, usually does not show before the age of 4 years. Since the triggers of perennial allergic rhinitis are constantly in the environment, it develops more quickly; its symptoms can appear as early as 18 months of age.

Symptoms

Table 10 lists the major symptoms of allergic rhinitis.

With either seasonal or perennial allergic rhinitis, the telltale symptom is repetitive sneezing; the unfortunate victim may reel off one sneeze after another, up to 20 or more in a brief period. This incessant, violent sneezing can quickly make the diaphragm, chest, and abdominal muscles tender and painful.

Causes

Allergic rhinitis is brought on by airborne allergens. Plant pollens (microscopic grains of protein material important to plant reproduction) cause hay fever. Determining which one or ones are to blame is fairly easy, and is tied to the pollenation cycle of a limited number and type of plants. Grasses usually pollenate only in the spring; trees pollenate in the late winter and early spring; weeds pollenate throughout the summer and into the fall. Thus, if your child's symptoms begin in the very early spring and last for a brief period of time, chances are that tree pollen is involved. Appendix E, a pollen calendar and chart, will help you pin down likely offenders in your area.

Perennial allergic rhinitis is caused by breathing in molds, house dust (often containing dust mites and cockroach particles), or animal danders, especially those of cats and horses. There are skin tests and newer blood tests available that will enable your doctor and you to identify the specific agent more exactly. Where the causes of the allergy are not absolutely clear and unmistakable, skin testing is a routine step in identifying the agent or agents responsible for your child's allergic rhinitis.

Skin Tests

Respiratory infections in children are so common and near-chronic that there is an understandable tendency to regard them as allergic in origin and to launch an expensive (and, in the end, unproductive) series of skin tests to identify the presumed causal agents. Skin tests should always be preceded by a complete, careful history and a scrupulous physical examination, which may be all that is required to account for the stubborn symptoms.

First Aid and Home Treatment of Hay Fever

Assuming that the diagnosis is accurate and its cause positively identified, first aid for and treatment of your child's allergic rhinitis has two components: (1) Help your child avoid altogether or reduce exposure to the cause or causes of the symptoms. This can often be accomplished simply by installing air-purification equipment in the bedroom and seeing to it that the child has as little contact with the allergens as can be managed. (If a pet is responsible for the condition, for instance, it should not have entry to the

Table 10
Symptoms of Allergic Rhinitis or Hay Fever

1.	Repetitive sneezing, worse in the morning
2.	An itch in the palate, throat, or ears
3.	Dark circles or allergic shiners under the eyes
4.	Itchy, watery eyes
5.	Nasal stuffiness
6.	A thin, watery mucus discharge from the nose
7.	Feeling a persistent need to scratch or wrinkle the nose
8.	Recurrent and unexplained nosebleeds
9.	Loss of the sense of taste

house and certainly not to the child's room; if pollen is the villain, keep the youngster inside and quiet on high pollen-count days.) Chapter 6 presents strategies to follow to avoid and control airborne allergens.

Parents sometimes ask about the advisability and effectiveness of moving away from a particular locality to escape a particular pollen. Even if the economic and social costs are disregarded, this is still a risky business, because the new location may have other vegetation that will trigger the allergic reaction. If the cause of the seasonal reaction is definitely known and the resources are available, relocating temporarily during the height of the pollen season sometimes helps.

Joyce, who is 9 and lives in Davenport, Iowa, has been miserable the past three summers. During August and September she suffered acutely from severe hay fever, which slipped into moderate asthma on occasion. Ragweed caused her distress. This year her family spent their vacation along the southern edge of Lake Superior, leaving in early August. Joyce and her mother stayed on at the Lake until Davenport had its first frost. This usually marks the end of the ragweed season. This year it happened in early September. Joyce missed the first week of school, but she did not mind missing the hay fever, which she avoided completely this year.

(2) Medicate, as necessary, after seeing your doctor. Table 11 lists the common treatment approaches to mild to severe hay fever. Table 12 lists the medications available and the ages at which they may be safely administered. The treatment of hay fever is almost always successful if done correctly and if the child takes the medicine as prescribed.

For mild, seasonal hay fever, antihistamines are the mainstay of treatment. They work by counteracting the histamine, which is released when antigens (pollens, and so on) invade the respiratory system. They have several serious drawbacks; the older drugs have a pronounced sedative effect, making the user drowsy and torpid, they sometimes cause gastric upsets or

Table 11
Treatment for Hay Fever Symptoms

Type of Symptoms	Treatment(s)	Comment
Mild, seasonal	Establish and avoid cause	Allergy Finder (Fig. I, Chapter 2) may help
	Use antihistamines as necessary	Avoid sedative over-the-counter antihistamines
Mild, perennial (year-round)	Establish and avoid cause	See above
	Invoke any necessary environmental controls	Air purifiers or conditioners can help greatly; other measures aimed at blocking out or minimizing exposure to allergens also extremely useful
	Use antihistamines as necessary	See above
	If symptoms not helped by antihistamines, ask physician for prescription for intranasal steroids or Nasalcrom	Must be taken at least a week before they affect symptoms
		Establish and use only minimum effective dose
		Avoid activities or environments that intensify symptoms
Moderate to severe, seasonal or perennial	Establish and avoid cause	See above
	Invoke any necessary environmental controls	See above
	Use prescription medications	See above
	Get allergy shots	If allergen has been positively identified and if indicated
	Reduce exposure by limiting activities appropriately	

complaints, and they often make children irritable or even hyperirritable. Because of this sedation, we do not recommend over-the-counter antihistamines. Claritin and Zyrtec, both once-per-day drugs, are relatively new antihistamines and can be very helpful. Zyrtec is the less expensive and more potent, but can cause sedation in a minority of people. If taken at night, however, Zyrtec is readily tolerated and very helpful. Both are available as liquids for young children. We do not recommend Seldane or Hismanal, because they risk causing sudden death. (These two drugs, if taken to excess or combined with other drugs, such as erythromycin, can cause a fatal cardiac arrythmia.)

For more severe or stubborn cases of allergic rhinitis, your physician may prescribe either intranasal synthetic steroids, or intranasal cromolyn sodium.

The management of hay fever depends on the age of the child and the length of the allergy season. For infants under 2 years of age, chronic runny noses are almost always owing to colds. In the very young child, it is more appropriate to establish the cause of the runny nose positively, and then take whatever steps are necessary to manage and reduce its complications.

Allergic rhinitis begins to show up in the young child from age 4 to 8 with the symptoms growing more severe over time as the sensitivity to the allergen increases. For children who have mild to moderate symptoms lasting no more than 4 to 6 weeks, the usual procedure is to prescribe antihistamines, forewarning the parents of their sedative side effects.

Where the symptoms are severe or prolonged, intranasal steroids (Beconase, Vancenase, Nasalide, Flonase, Rhinocort, Nasalcort) virtually always work; if they do not, the diagnosis of allergic rhinitis may be wrong. Intranasal steroids are not approved for children under 6, although it is not unusual for doctors to prescribe them for somewhat younger children who are severely allergic. Administered as a nasal spray, they carry a cortisone-like medication. There is hardly any absorption of the medication so that cortisone's negative side effects are avoided. Intranasal steroids are extremely effective; for children with severe hay fever, they are almost always the preferred treatment and they are far superior to anything else available. Intranasal steroids are preventive measures; to be maximally effective, they must be started before symptoms appear and continued without fail during the entire allergy season. They can, however, produce nosebleeds. Many of these sprays come in an aqueous formulation, which is often better tolerated.

We do not advocate the use of either oral steroids (such as pills) or injectable steroids (steroid "shots") for the treatment of allergic rhinitis. Not long ago, it was fairly common to administer a 5- or 7-day course of prednisone or another cortisone by mouth at the peak of allergy season. This was before the days of intranasal steroids. It was also common for people to get injections of a long-acting steroid known as Celestone. Both of these tactics are unnecessary and may be dangerous. The long-term use of steroids can cause osteoporosis, a condition that causes the bones to thin; they may induce cataracts in the eyes or bring about destruction of the hip joint, a disease known as aseptic necrosis, or even increase the likelihood of contracting serious infections. Thus, for a problem as mild as hay fever, it is unnecessary to use oral or injectable steroids. On the other hand, intranasal steroids do not carry these side effects and, if used strictly as prescribed, may be safely taken over a period of years. For many allergy sufferers, the advent of these preparations has been a godsend.

Mark, now 12, developed hay fever when he was 5. He lives in a rural part of northern California, and he is especially sensitive to indigenous grasses and weeds. Over the years, his mother, who is determinedly New Age and antiestablishment, has had Mark treated by a succession of local herbalists and other nontraditional healers—to no avail. Each successive spring and summer his symptoms worsened and, finally, when Mark was 10, became so severe that the mother grudgingly took him to the local clinic. The doctor in attendance there prescribed Flonase, instructed him on how to take it, two sprays in each nostril once a day, told him he would not feel any better for 5 days, but afterward things would improve. Five days later, his stuffy, scratchy, itchy, irritable nose and throat began to clear up, and 2 weeks after starting the medication, it was as if he had never had any symptoms at all.

For the severely allergic child who gets side effects from intranasal steroids, there is intranasal cromolyn sodium (Nasalcrom). Also a preventive measure, it has been available in the United States for several years. Administered as a nasal spray, it is effective in children as young as 4 years without causing irritation to their nasal membranes as intranasal steroids sometimes do, nor does it carry antihistamine's sedative side effects. Nasalcrom is generally not as effective as intranasal steroids. Sometimes these two types of sprays can be used in concert for severe or otherwise nonresponsive youngsters.

There is a special word that must be said about decongestants. Decongestants are widely used in over-the-counter medications and are found in most cold medicines. By far their most common ingredient is pseudoephedrine, commonly known as Sudafed. Why these drugs have continued to enjoy such popularity is a mystery; perhaps it is because they have been around so long that no one has really troubled to examine them carefully and critically. Almost all of them are available over-the-counter. There is no convincing evidence that the oral decongestants work at all and the decongestant nasal sprays like Afrin and 4-Way among many others carry nasty side effects.

The use of these sprays may temporarily reduce the swelling in the nose and make your child feel better momentarily. However, after using one or another of them for more than a few days at a time, the nose actually becomes addicted to it, and a disease known as rhinitis medicamentosa develops. This leads to swelling and clogging of the nasal membranes, called turbinates. The swelling can be so bad that the child is unable to breathe and uses even more nasal spray. In time, the child may be taking nasal spray 20 or more times a day.

Rhinitis medicamentosa is a disease that can be even more serious than hay fever. Treating this problem requires that the decongestants be stopped. In the first stages and in mild cases, the doctor would prescribe the intranasal steroids we discussed above. In more serious cases, a more potent intranasal spray known as decadron turbinaire would probably be called in. Decadron turbinaire was widely used as an intranasal steroid before the newer sprays

Table 12
Medications for Allergic Rhinitis for Use at Given Ages

MEDICATIONS	AGE			
	Under 2	2-6	6-12	Over 12
Over-the-Counter[a]				
Antihistamines				
Actifed	No	Yes	Yes	Yes
Chlortrimetron	No	Yes	Yes	Yes
Prescription				
Antihistamines				
Zyrtec	No	No	Yes	Yes
Claritin	No	No	Yes	Yes
Intranasal Steroids				
Beconase	No	No	No	Yes
Vancenase	No	No	No	Yes
Nasalide	No	No	Yes	Yes
Flonase	No	No	Yes	Yes
Rhinocort	No	No	Yes	Yes
Nasalcort	No	No	Yes	Yes
Intranasal cromolyn sodium				
Nasalcrom	No	Yes	Yes	Yes
Intranasal decongestants	DO NOT USE—SEE PAGE 108			
Afrin				
Neosynephrine				
4-Way				

[a]NOT recommended because of sedation.

came out. However, it can be absorbed by the body, and it can carry some of the same side effects as cortisone taken by mouth. Accordingly, except for this condition, it is very rarely used. For the most stubborn cases of rhinitis medicamentosa, it may be necessary to give cortisone by mouth for several days or longer to allow the nasal membranes to shrink. After they have shrunk, intranasal steroids can be begun. Rhinitis medicimentosa can be a very unpleasant disease to have and is often extremely difficult to treat. Accordingly, shun using intranasal decongestants in treating your child's nasal problems.

Long-Term Treatment

Long-term treatment of allergic rhinitis has three elements:

1. Constant, unrelenting avoidance or control of the triggers that precipitate attacks. This is the most important precaution you can take, and it is one that you must impress on your child.

2. Appropriate use of medication.
3. Where indicated, desensitization (allergy shots).

In children whose symptoms persist for longer periods or are year-round, allergy shots may be effective. We strongly believe that only allergists should give or prescribe allergy shots. There are many nonallergists who administer shots, but if you live in an area where one is available, we strongly urge you to consult with or get a second opinion from a board-certified allergist.

Jill has been having a chronic runny nose for the past 4 years. Her mother took her to Dr. Honald, a well-regarded ear, nose, and throat specialist who does some allergy on the side. He has not taken an allergy course in many years and, like many physicians, has not kept current with the recent developments in immunology. He treated Jill with allergy shots for her chronic runny nose. Her nasal symptoms improved with the shots, but her mother noted that her eczema, which had been mild, worsened. Dr. Honald did not believe that the symptoms were related, but at the mother's insistence, referred the child to an allergist. The allergist knew that allergy shots in children with eczema can make the skin become worse. She stopped the shots, and prescribed intranasal steroids instead. The nasal symptoms cleared up, and so did Jill's skin after the shots were stopped.

Complications

Runny noses result from a number of conditions that can lead to a misdiagnosis of allergic rhinitis.

Upper respiratory infections (colds) are sometimes difficult to distinguish from allergic rhinitis, although an infection is usually at fault if:

Fever is present;
The nasal discharge is thick, yellow, or pus-like; or
The mucous tissue has a characteristic, boggy appearance.

Colds are often mistaken for allergies because colds are so prevalent in small children. Many parents complain that their preschoolers have runny noses all of the time and the near-chronic infection can lead to the false conclusion that an allergy is to blame. In young children, colds are especially problematic when child day care centers are in the picture or older children bring colds home. Chapters 5 and 20 tell you how you can decrease expo- sure to and minimize the severity of respiratory infections.

Vasomotor rhinitis sometimes occurs in children. The chief complaint in vasomotor rhinitis is a chronic runny nose, often made worse by cold, heat, or exercise. A careful examination by your doctor can usually establish that it is vasomotor rhinitis and not the result of an allergy. Patients are often misdiagnosed as having allergic rhinitis and given an ineffective course of antiallergy treatment. Help can be found, however, by using a new intrana-sal spray, called Atrovent. This medicine blocks the production of the ex-cess fluid and works almost immediately. It is very good at treating this problem, but is associated with an uncomfortable feeling of dryness in the mouth and throat in some people.

Ear infections often accompany and are triggered by allergic rhinitis. *See* Chapter 16 for more about this common and troublesome condition.

Sinusitis is another fellow-traveler of nasal allergies or infections. The sinuses are cavities located behind the nose and below the eyes. Although their exact function is not clear, they and the nose are lined by the same tissue and they open into the nose by small openings known as sinus ostia, which allow the exchange of secretion produced in the sinuses. Anything that clogs the nose can block the sinuses, and the inflammation called sinusitis can result. Rare in children under 3 years of age, it produces a vari-ety of complaints—headaches, fever, a stuffy feeling at the back of the nose and under the eyes.

In children over 3, sinusitis may be a chronic and often undiagnosed prob-lem. It can only be confidently diagnosed with a CT scan. (Although we do *not* advocate that CT scans be administered routinely, where chronic sinusi-tis is a possibility, a four-way (four pictures) CT scan should be done; a single picture can confirm the diagnosis of sinusitis and, if it is present, point to appropriate treatment.)

13

Eczema and Dry Skin

Even though we teach our children that "Beauty is only skin deep," our society so values clear, flawless skin that billions of dollars are spent each year on the hundreds of skin lotions, creams, cleansers, conditioners, and cover-ups that crowd drugstore shelves. Because of this attitude, skin problems—including those resulting from allergic skin disorders—cause considerable grief, much of which is avoidable.

The skin is an amazingly resilient organ. Left alone or given the right kind of help, it often recovers completely from the most severe damage. This is especially true for allergic skin disorders whose lesions almost always clear up without a trace.

Incidence

Eczema affects about four children in 100. It is slightly more common in girls, but occurs equally often in the various racial or ethnic groups in the United States. It is more prevalent in urban, industrialized localities. If either parent has a history of hay fever, asthma, or eczema, the probability of eczema in the child increases substantially. While mainly a problem in infants, eczema can manifest itself at any age and in somewhat different forms as Table 13 spells out.

Dry skin (which is usually observed in children with eczema, although the reverse is not true) is a minor but annoying condition that can generally be managed without incident by following the procedures listed in Table 14.

Usual Age of Onset

The majority of children with eczema develop it in infancy, somewhere between the second and twelfth month of life; approx 90% of its victims turn up with the symptoms before they reach the age of 5. The remaining 10% develop it in later childhood or even as adults.

Table 13
Classification of Eczema

Stage	Type of lesion	Usual sites of lesion	Other associated symptoms
Infant (2 months– 2 years)	Dry, chapped skin, which gives way to red, inflamed areas made up of small blisters: scratching leads to crusting and oozing	Cheeks, spreading to forehead, scalp, ears, trunk, and extremities	Irritability and sleeplessness
Childhood (2–12 years)	Red, inflamed areas of small blisters, which are enlarged and encrusted by scratching; drier than in infant stage	Inside elbows and back of knees; ear lobes and behind ears	Dry skin; anxiousness; irritability; hyperactivity
Adolescent and adult (over 12 years)	Large, thickened areas of skin surrounded by crusted blisters	Insides of elbows and knees; eyelids, wrists hands, feet	Dry skin; prominent profuse "goose bumps"

Symptoms

Regardless of the stage of life at which it turns up, eczema is accompanied by intense itching, which is its first, most prominent, and most distressing feature. The itching precedes the appearance of lesions, which take slightly different forms and blossom on different parts of the body, depending on the age at which they first appear.

Causes

We do not definitely know the cause or causes of eczema. Onset or worsening of symptoms has been linked to some foods, to airborne allergens—pollens, house dust, molds, animal dander—and to psychological stress.

Foods and Eczema

Carefully conducted experiments using skin tests that tried to tie hypersensitivity to specific foods to eczema have proven inconclusive. In any case, routine skin testing for individuals suffering from eczema is not recommended because of the risk of triggering a reaction or worsening an existing one. Thus, all that can be said about eczema symptoms is that they are associated or linked with other bodily signs of allergy and are quite pos-

Table 14
First Aid and Home Treatment for Eczema

1. Check for infection. If serious scratch marks, widespread lesions, significant crusting, or severe discoloration are present, *See a physician today.* (Infections are common with eczema, and antibiotics are the usual and effective means of treatment.)
2. To control itching, scratching, and spread of lesions
   —Keep fingernails trimmed as short as possible
   —Avoid activities causing excessive sweating or emotional stress
   —*Do not* wear tight or overly warm clothing
   —*Do not* wear wool or other harsh fabrics
   —Avoid temperature extremes
   —Avoid harsh soaps, detergents, and petrochemicals (Dove is recommended as a mild soap. *Do not* use Ivory since it is very irritating to eczema).
   —Apply protective dressings and, if necessary, protective cuffs in the case of infants and small children
   —Apply Burow's solution to the "wet" type of lesion (Burow's solution, aluminum acetate, is available over-the-counter at the pharmacy). Follow directions for preparation and application strictly.
3. If the foregoing remedies do not give relief, consult a physician who will likely prescribe corticosteroid creams or ointments, which are effective for control or spread of lesions, and antihistamines, which probably because of their sedative effect, sometimes relieve itching and scratching.
4. About bathing, opinion is divided. We believe bathing where the "dry" type of eczema is involved should be limited to two or three times per week. Leisurely baths (30 min or more) in tepid water are recommended. Nonlanolin-based oils and nonirritating soaps, such as Dove, should be used. A lotion applied to the body after bathing soothes and relieves itching and prevents excessive drying of skin. Use nonwater-based cleansers like Cetaphil between baths.
5. Elimination diets, which take account of suspected food irritants, should be instituted and followed strictly for at least 2 weeks (*see* Appendix A for detailed instructions).
6. Other suspected irritants should be controlled as much as possible (*see* Chapter 8 for advice).
7. Allergy shots are usually to be avoided because of the danger of provoking a reaction and because eczema does not respond especially well to this form of treatment.

sibly made worse by exposure to allergy-producing substances to which the individual is susceptible—foods, dust and pollens, animal dander, molds. Consequently, the sufferers or their parents must rely on elimination diets (*see* Chapter 4) or careful, critical observations to identify the agents that appear to produce or worsen the symptoms. Because of the possible role of foods in provoking eczema, it is strongly recommended that newborn children with allergic parents be breast-fed for at least their first 6 months. This will delay the need to feed babies formula, cow's milk, and other foods until later in the first year of life. Breast-fed babies whether of allergic or nonallergic parents, have less eczema (indeed, fewer allergies of all kinds) than bottle-fed babies.

The treatment of eczema has to take into account a number of factors—type and extent of the disease, age and occupation of the victim, presence or absence of infection. The steps to follow in seeking help or relief are outlined below.

First Aid and Home Treatment of Eczema

Home treatment of eczema has two aspects: controlling the itching and caring for the lesions. What you will do depends to some extent on the age of your child. Follow the steps in Table 14. In older sufferers with chronic, stubborn eczema, three to four brief exposures per week to UV light (sunlight) can relieve mild or moderate symptoms. Avoid sunburn!

> Wes, a teenager, learned the hard way that too much sun can add up to disaster. He heard that psoriasis, another skin disease, is helped by sunlight. Accordingly he bought a sunlamp, used the protective glasses as advised, and gradually acclimated his skin to increasing exposure over a 7-day period. By the week's end, he was using it 1 hour per day. Within 2 weeks, his skin was dry and itchy. After three weeks his skin was an inflamed mess.

Long-Term Treatment

If you follow the procedures covered in Table 14 faithfully, your child's eczema will usually respond to them. If the symptoms persist, become worse, or the lesions become infected, see your pediatrician or family practitioner at once. In addition, take steps to identify and avoid any substances that are associated with the appearance or worsening of symptoms. Foods (milk, eggs, wheat, legumes, fish, potatoes) and airborne antigens (pollens, mold, dust, animal dander) are the most common offenders (*see* Chapters 4 and 6). Skin tests can help to pin down the allergens associated with eczema, but they should be used cautiously because they can trigger eczema symptoms.

Finally, try to create an atmosphere that is free of psychological stress for your child by concentrating on doing specific things to relieve the discomfort.

Do not try to control scratching by nagging or punishing the child. Such actions will not relieve the fierce itching, and may simply focus attention on the complaint rather than persuading or making it possible for the child to leave the itchy spots alone.

Duration

In infants, eczema usually clears up without complications or any damage to the skin by the time the child turns 4. In older children and adolescents, the symptoms may persist—in about one-fifth of cases into adulthood—but they become more localized and usually respond to medication. The lesions can be quite unsightly, and the temptation to mask them with cosmetics should be avoided, since many cosmetics contain substances which actually bring on the symptoms or make them worse.

Complications

Infections: Eczema lesions, because of the nearly irresistible temptation to scratch them, often develop secondary infections. Infections are usually treated with and respond to antibiotics, although antibiotic salves containing neomycin should be avoided in treating secondary infections of eczema.

Herpes simplex (fever blisters, cold sores): A herpes infection in a person with eczema can spread rapidly to cover much of the body and presents a serious threat. If eczema is accompanied or followed by a herpes infection, see your doctor immediately.

Special Hints

Although eczema lesions are unsightly, they are not "catching" and you need not fear body contact with a child with eczema. It is perfectly safe for people with eczema to prepare or handle food and to have ordinary forms of contact with others.

Efamol (oil of evening primrose) is often recommended for treatment of eczema. The evidence indicates that it is not particularly effective with young children, but in adolescents and adults it does help. It has two drawbacks. First, it is quite expensive. Second, over-the-counter imitations of Efamol, which are available in health food stores, differ chemically from the prescription version, and their effectiveness has not been proven.

14

Hives

Incidence

Hives, known medically as urticaria, are the most common allergic or hypersensitivity reaction found in children. One person in five will have hives at one time or another.

Usual Age of Onset

Hives can crop up at any age. Children are especially likely to develop hives after eating certain foods or in conjunction with viral infections.

Symptoms

Hives are blotchy patches of red, slightly elevated skin (wheals), which blanch or whiten when touched. The lesions, which can range in size from quite small to several inches in diameter, may cover much of the body in severe cases. They are usually intensely itchy, especially when located in areas covered by hair or in the webs of toes and fingers.

The *acute* form of the disorder follows release of histamine by the body's mast cells. This release of histamine may trigger a variety of reactions, one of which is the hive lesions.

Onset of the acute form of hives may be dramatically swift with symptoms showing within minutes of exposure to a causal agent. Because of this narrow time gap between exposure and display of symptoms, it is often possible to make a hard and fast identification of the substance causing the outbreak.

The original wheals fade rapidly, ordinarily within the space of a few hours, but they also tend to migrate, relocating on other parts of the body. Where there is no additional exposure, the symptoms customarily clear within a day or two, and they rarely persist for more than a week.

Causes

Often the symptoms so closely follow exposure to a trigger that the cause is obvious.

Dan, 12, goes to a neighborhood park with a group of his friends for a game of touch football. During the course of the contest, he takes off his shoes to improve his footing and, not long after that, steps on a bee, which stings him. Within a few minutes, he develops a mild case of hives, intensely itchy wheals on his legs and in the groin area. By this time, the foot that has been stung has swollen to the point where he is unable to put his shoe back on so he has to hobble home barefoot. When he gets home, his father calls the doctor who tells them what to do to counter the pain, swelling, and itching, and also informs them that this sort of reaction to a bee sting has serious implications. He says that Dan should be kept under observation for an hour or so and brought in to the office soon for a consultation. Dan's hives fade quickly, and by the next morning he is clear of them, although the site of the bee sting is still tender and quite itchy.

Table 15 names the types of agents that most often provoke hives in children, and lists a few of the many specific substances or conditions that produce them.

Hives may show up as part of a more general or systemic reaction with anaphylactic shock being a possibility. *Consequently, the appearance of hives should act as a signal to watch closely for the appearance of other possibly lethal signs.*

In the acute form, the lesions usually clear up without incident in a day or two; if they persist for more than six weeks, the condition is termed chronic. What provokes the chronic form of the complaint is much more difficult to establish, since histamine release does not seem to play a role. As a consequence, the search for the precipitating cause may be long, difficult, and in about 70–80% of cases, unsuccessful.

Hives can also be associated with a number of chronic diseases, including hyperthyroidism, systemic lupus erythematosus, juvenile rheumatoid arthritis, lymphoma, and some cancers. Checking the thyroid gland function is an important step in treatment. Sometimes patients with unremitting hives are found to have antithyroid antibodies, but normal thyroid function. Interestingly, these people may respond to taking thyroid replacement.

As with most other allergic reactions, the underlying causes or mechanisms that produce hives remain unknown.

Treatment of Hives

Although hives usually vanish after a short period of time, leaving only the memory of blemishes and acute discomfort from the itching, they should be watched closely for two reasons: They may be associated with serious or

Table 15
Triggers for Hives in Children*

Category	Principal offenders
Food	Eggs, peanuts, nuts, chocolate, berries, seafood, tomatoes, milk, cheese, yeast
Food additives	Tartrazine, benzoates
Drugs	Penicillin, aspirin, and sulfonamides especially; almost all other drugs possible
Insects	Bites, stings, body material
Inhalants (rarely)	Pollens, dust, mold, animal dander
Infections	Viral infections, parasitic infestations, hepatitis, abscessed teeth
Systemic disease	Rheumatic disorders, hyperthyroidism, certain malignancies
Psychological factors	Extremes of tension, stress, anxiety

*There are also several special physical causes of hives or urticaria, which are described in Table 16.

even life-threatening complications, which require drastic emergency treatment, and they sometimes accompany chronic, noninfectious diseases. The mainstay of treatment is the use of antihistamines to reduce itching. Sadly, although antihistamines are often effective, they almost always induce severe sedation.

> Lauren, a middle-school student with recurring bouts of hives, could predict her school grades by the amount of antihistamines she took—the higher the dose, the lower her test scores. Fortunately, her doctor found out that Lauren's hives could be controlled by Zyrtec, a new, potent antihistamine with much less sedative properties.

Skin testing and courses of allergy shots are generally not recommended for treatment of hives. First aid and home treatment measures for treatment of hives appear in Table 17.

Long-Term Treatment

Acute hives rarely persist for more than a few days. If they hang on for longer than 48 hours or if they resist treatment, see your doctor. The doctor may try different types of antihistamines from the mild over-the-counter drugs, such as Chlortrimetron, to potent very sedative-inducing drugs, such as Benadryl, Atarax, and Vistaril. The new antihistamine Zyrtec can be very helpful. It is effective when taken only once per day, but does have a sedative effect on some people. Be sure to discuss this with your doctor. On occasion, tranquilizers, such as Sinequan, may be used. Although Sinequan does have antianxiety properties, it is an extremely potent antihistamine. Control of anxiety can also help reduce the itching and, therefore, the hives. Thus, Sinequan is often effective. However, there is little evidence that hives are psychologically induced.

Table 16
Physical Urticarias—Recognition, Avoidance, Treatment

Name[a]	Cause and symptoms	Avoidance or control strategies	Treatment
Dermographism	Wheals in response to firm stroking of the skin		Antihistamines
Pressure urticaria	Red, deep, local painful swelling sometime after skin is exposed to sustained pressure (as of shoes, belts, and so on)	Relieve pressure	Does not respond to antihistamine. Low dosage of prednisone helpful
Cold-induced	Burny, itchy eruption, headache, wheezing, fainting within minutes of exposure to cold	Dress warmly, warm gradually	Desensitize to prevent urticaria wheezing triggered by exposure to cold. A drug called Periactin is often very effective
Heat-induced urticaria	Wheals after contact with heated object or hot bath or shower	Avoid heat	Antihistamines (if necessary)
Cholinergic urticaria	Small wheals (1–2 mm) surrounded by larger inflamed red patches associated with elevated core body temperature (i.e., following exercise, bathing)	Take medication before exercise	Antihistamines
Solar urticaria	Itchy red patches within minutes of exposure to sun or artificial light	Use a sunscreen	Antihistamines

[a]This table lists only the most common causes of physical urticaria in children. There are many other substances or factors which are known or thought to trigger hives although they are rarely encountered in practice.

Table 17
Treatment of Hives (acute type with sudden onset)

1. *Take oral antihistamines* (Benadryl, Chlortrimetron [both over the counter] or the pre-scription drugs Atarax or Zyrtec) for lesions and relief of itching.
2. *Keep victim quiet for at least 30 minutes* and watch closely for additional reactions. *Any of the following, if they appear, require that the individual receive emergency medical treatment at once. If necessary, summon the fire department, rescue squad,or ambulance.*

Difficulty with breathing	Constricted feeling in chest
Abdominal pain	Wheezing
Difficulty in swallowing	Nausea or vomiting
Weakness	Hoarseness or thickened speech
Confusion	Drop in blood pressure
Bluish or purplish coloration	Collapse
Irregular or thready pulse	Unconsciousness
Incontinence	

3. *If hives alone worsen or persist for more than 48 hours*, see a physician as soon as possible. (The physician will take a history and may order laboratory tests to try to pinpoint causes and, *most important*, rule out the possibility that other, more serious diseases or infections are responsible for the reaction.)
4. *Avoid* vasodilators including alcohol, aspirin, heat, exertion, and emotional stress.
5. *Avoid* quinine, opiates (codeine, meperidine, morphine), antibiotics (chlortetracycline, polymyxins), and certain vitamins (thiamine), which can directly release allergic mediators from mast cells.
6. To control itching (additional measures)
   Take tepid water baths to which Aveeno colloidal oatmeal has been added.
   Apply cool or ice compresses.
   Use itch suppressing lotions, such as 0.25% menthol 1% phenol in calamine lotion (Eucerin), Schamberg's lotion, or Caladryl.
7. It is *rarely* necessary to use cortisone in the treatment of hives, although it is sometimes helpful for severe *acute* urticaria, pressure urticaria, or severe, chronic urticaria.

For very severe cases of chronic hives, your doctor may also prescribe Cimetidine, a drug that has generally been used to treat the acidity associated with ulcers. Finally, for chronic relentless cases, steroids may be used, although we try to avoid them whenever possible because of their serious side effects.

Angioedema

Angioedema, which is often associated with hives, may occur as single or multiple and widespread lesions. Unlike hives, however, its nonpitting, sharply demarcated, and *nonitching* swellings may crop up at any place on or in the body. Lesions of angioedema, like those of hives, may be of short duration, but if they do persist, they migrate every 24 to 48 hours. In angioedema (*angio*-blood; *edema*-swelling), the soft tissues around the eyes,

Table 18
First Aid and Treatment for Angioedema

1. If red, raised, *nonitching* lesions on the surface of the skin are present, administer antihistamines like Benadryl or Atarax.
2. If mucous or soft tissue is affected, *watch closely for additional symptoms*. If any of the following appear, seek emergency treatment at once. If necessary, summon fire department, rescue squad, or ambulance.

   Difficulty with breathing
   Difficulty in swallowing
   Abdominal pain
   Constricted feeling in throat or chest
   Hoarseness or thickened speech

* *

   After Initial Attack:
3. See a physician (allergist) as soon as possible for diagnostic tests and medical treatment of the hereditary form of the disorder if it is found, or medical control of the acquired form.
4. Avoid any known precipitating causes.
5. Avoid the following possible precipitating causes.

   Trauma or physical injury
   Dusts and pollens
   Strenuous, taxing exercise
   Extremes of cold
   Vibration
   Pressure
6. Carry and know how to use a kit for anaphylactic emergencies. (Get a prescription for an ANA-KIT from your doctor.)
7. Wear a Medic-Alert bracelet, appropriately inscribed.

the lips, and the genitals are often involved, and the gastrointestinal and pulmonary tracts may be affected. Swelling in the larynx, which sometimes occurs, is dangerous and, in rare instances, fatal, causing death by asphyxiation.

About 10% of the population may experience both hives and angioedema; hives alone will be seen in 8% and angioedema alone will affect 2% of the population. For unknown reasons, angioedema occurs more frequently in women 40 to 49 years of age; it is uncommon in children.

In almost three-quarters of cases, the precipitating cause of angioedema is unknown. Moreover, there is no reliable way to diagnose angioedema with laboratory tests. One exception to this statement is a rare familial angioedema known as hereditary angioneurotic edema. (The allergist is often in the awkward position of having to say, "You've got so and so, but I cannot tell you what is causing it." This is especially true for angioedema.)

There are good reasons for getting a confirmed diagnosis of angioedema. First, the disorder comes in two forms, one acquired and one inherited or genetically transmitted. Individuals having *hereditary* angioedema can be treated medically so as to minimize the risk and the severity of attacks.

Second, in either its hereditary or acquired form, angioedema is potentially life-threatening, and individuals having the disorder should be aware of its existence. They should also know what steps to take in the event of an attack and wear Medic-Alert identification so that others will also know of and be able to respond swiftly and appropriately in an emergency.

Attacks of angioedema have been associated with the following conditions:

Trauma or injury (especially to soft tissue of the upper respiratory tract, such as occurs in tooth extraction or tonsillectomy).
Heavy exposure to inhalant allergens (dusts or pollens).
Strenuous exercise.
Cold.
Vibration.
Pressure.
Use of birth control pills.

First aid and treatment for children diagnosed as susceptible to angioedema are given in Table 18.

15

Itchy Eyes

Everyone, at some time or another, has probably had red, itchy eyes. There are scores of reasons for itchy eyes but dirt and foreign material or objects in the eye are most commonly responsible. The pharmaceutical industry, in contrast, has long recognized the economic possibilities that appear in red, inflamed eyes; drugstore shelves are filled with generally worthless eyedrops. Following are accounts of four children who were taken to allergists because of suspected allergies. All had similar symptoms, but a vastly different diagnosis.

Bob, 11 plays left field for his little league baseball team. No matter what he seems to do his eyes get red during games. His mother is convinced that he is allergic to his baseball glove. His doctor is convinced there is nothing wrong with him. His father is convinced that it is all in his head. Bob knows it gets worse during the daytime, whenever he looks into the sun and especially when he is out there in the field, staring intently, waiting for a ball to be hit to him. As it happens, Bob's eyes are simply very sensitive to sunlight, which causes them to water copiously. As they water, Bob rubs them to clear his vision. The process of rubbing produced a simple nonallergic irritation. Sunglasses were all he needed to clean up the problem.

Doe, 13, is taken to her doctor because she has severely swollen, red, and itchy eyelids. Her mother is convinced her problems are from using eye makeup. In this case, Mom has it right. Doe is allergic to some of the chemicals in the makeup, which are very, very irritating to her tender skin.

Paul, 12, gets severely itchy eyes every spring—they become so swollen that he can barely see. He often has chronic repetitive sneezing at the same time. His eyes almost always get worse on a windy day or when the newspaper forecasts a high pollen count. Paul has classic hay fever and allergic conjunctivitis. His treatment, avoidance and eyedrops containing antihistamines, is extremely effective.

Charley's dad is a house painter who carries all of his materials—paints, brushes, turpentine, ladders, and so forth,—in the back of the family van. Charley's eyes begin to water as soon as he gets in the vehicle. His dad thought it was owing to an allergy to the vinyl upholstery. He could not believe it could be from the paint and the fumes because Charley, 10, had been riding in the van for years without any problem. Nonetheless, problems, habits, and irritations change, and his son's watery eyes are in fact owing to fumes.

Doe and Paul's are allergic reactions; Bob and Charley's are simple irritations.

Incidence

Allergic conjunctivitis, chronically red and itching eyes, is a common problem in children. It usually accompanies hay fever.

Usual Age of Onset

Allergic conjunctivitis usually shows up in 4-to-6 year-olds, although it may appear at any age thereafter. It often begins in spring or is associated with having a pet, particularly a cat. If your child has never had any allergies and then begins to develop eye symptoms after age 16, the symptoms are probably not allergic although, as in everything else in life, there are some exceptions.

Kevin, now 17, lived in Detroit, Michigan until last year when his family moved to Dodge City, Kansas. Kevin had no allergies in Detroit, but within the first year after settling in Dodge City, Kevin began to complain that his eyes and his ears itched. Also, he noticed that in the morning, he sneezed uncontrollably seven or eight times in a row. His parents could not understand why, out of the blue, Kevin suddenly developed allergies. What they did not realize is that Kevin had moved out of the cement city into farm—and pollen—country.

Symptoms

Allergic conjunctivitis is usually bilateral, that is, it involves both eyes. They will be red and itchy and will worsen with rubbing. The itching and inflammation will vary in intensity with location. They will usually be worse out-of-doors if the offending agent is pollen, or indoors if the offending agent is house dust or animal dander.

If the child has involvement in only one eye, *Beware!* This might be a severe infection. See a doctor immediately.

The irritation, if it is owing to allergies, will virtually always appear about the same time as other allergies, particularly hay fever, crop up. Thus, it is unusual to have allergic eyes without also having an allergic runny nose, asthma, or some other allergic disease.

Causes

The causes of allergic conjunctivitis are the big five of allergies—tree pollen, grass pollen, weed pollen, house dust, and animal dander. Molds generally do not produce allergic conjunctivitis. By far the biggest offenders are grass pollen and animal dander. Grass pollen is a major cause simply because there is so much of it in the springtime and because children play out-of-doors and are exposed to it. Animal dander, an equally major problem, is prevalent indoors; it occurs because it is so easy to get animal dander on the fingers and transfer it to the eyes. Children also develop symptoms from picking up animal dander inadvertently.

> Brad, 9, has been visiting his grandmother's house virtually every Sunday since he was an infant. His mother has always known that he is allergic to his grandmother's dog, so she has him wash his hands thoroughly and cautions him not to rub his eyes whenever he is at her house. On a recent trip, the family put up at a motel in Oregon. Within 30 minutes of arriving in the room, Brad began to sneeze and to rub his eyes. His eyes were itching and tearing so badly that he was practically crying. His mother recognized his symptoms as being the same as the ones he got at grandma's house. Although there were no animals in the room, she came to realize later that many travelers bring dogs and cats into motel rooms—and motel housekeeping is often so haphazard that the animal dander would pile up from a succession of canine and feline guests.

When to See the Doctor

The biggest problem with allergic conjunctivitis is not the allergy itself, but the tendency to confuse it with other eye problems. Serious bacterial infections of the eye often mimic allergic conjunctivitis, and only a good examination by the doctor will pick up the difference. *This is not an exam that you should do.* This is because certain viral infections can closely resemble bacterial infections or allergic symptoms, and can be very severe. Adenovirus and herpes viruses, two frequent causes of eye irritation, are found everywhere on the body. All too often these viruses get in the child's eye. The parents may think an allergy is responsible because the viral symptoms closely resemble allergic ones. They respond by administering the same eye drops prescribed for allergic conjunctivitis. The trouble is that some of the eye drops designed to treat allergic conditions have steroids or cortisone in them; when these steroids are put into an infected eye, the disease can virtually explode, even bringing about blindness.

> Suzy, 11 has had allergic conjunctivitis for several years. The symptoms usually appear only during the months of May and June when the pollen count is high. However, in mid-November, not long after a cold, her mother noted that Suzy's eyes were quite red and teary. She assumed it was from her allergies, and she put eyedrops, containing steroids, in Suzy's eyes. These were the drops that the doctor had prescribed during springtime for Suzy. This time Suzy had an adenovirus infection of her eyes and the eyedrops caused a

severe reaction. Fortunately, the medication did not bring about significant impairment in vision, although it could easily have led to scarring of the cornea and total loss of vision.

Unless the symptoms are unmistakably and clearly familiar, and follow an established allergic pattern, *take all eye problems to your child's doctor.*

First Aid and Home Treatment of Itchy Eyes

The first thing to do in allergic conjunctivitis is establish the cause of the problem. Use the criteria and standards we have listed above to do this.

Second, identify the reason. Reviewing the questions in Fig. 6, a good checklist of the potential triggers, will help you do this.

Third, impose environmental controls to the fullest extent possible. See Chapter 6 for methods of controlling airborne allergens. Keep fingers out of eyes. Scratching and rubbing the eyes will only make the symptoms worse. Wash your child's hands if he or she has petted a dog or cat.

Fourth, apply ocular antihistamines, now available as over-the-counter eyedrops; these medications contain the same antihistamines used to treat hay fever. These are very effective in reducing the itching and the redness of allergic conjunctivitis. Since they are put into eyes, they do not produce the sedation that they do when taken by mouth although they can cause irritation in some susceptible persons and they can burn. Intraocular cromolyn, much like the cromolyn used for allergic rhinitis or asthma, is also available. It was popular in the early 1980s, but fell from favor when a contaminant was discovered in many bottles. It is now available from another company, and contamination is not an issue. Although expensive and no more effective, it is less irritating than antihistamines and is used by many patients for long-term treatment. There are a variety of other more potent drugs available as well. The medications used to treat allergic rhinitis and their advantages and disadvantages are listed in Table 19. In addition, Table 19 contains the names of over-the-counter eye medicines and eye washes that you can buy from your pharmacy. These over-the-counter drugs are relatively cheap, but are no substitute for an accurate diagnosis and proper treatment. They sometimes produce a soothing effect, perhaps by flushing away the pollen and dander in the eye. They are not a long-term remedy, however.

Fifth, children who have severe and chronic allergic conjunctivitis almost always show some other allergic symptom, such as hay fever. Accordingly, the use of oral medications to treat these symptoms will usually help the allergic conjunctivitis too.

Vernal Conjunctivitis

Vernal conjunctivitis refers to a specific type of eye irritation occurring mostly in the springtime—hence, the name vernal. Most commonly, it affects boys, although girls may also develop it. The onset of vernal con-

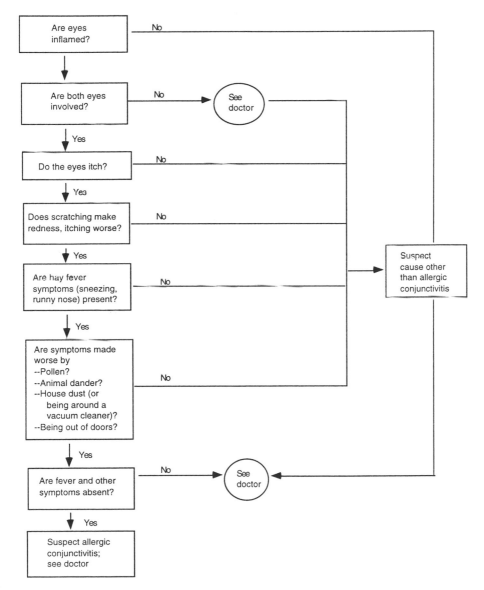

Fig. 6. Allergic conjunctivitis test questions.

Table 19
Eyedrops Used to Treat Allergic Conjunctivitis

Over-the-counter	Ingredients	Comment
Murine™; Visine	Decongestants	Reduces eye redness
Naphcon™	Antihistamine vasoconstrictor	Extremely effective but burns
Vasocon®	Antihistamine vasoconstrictor	Extremely effective but burns
Prescription		
Acular®	Ketorolac	Moderately effective if used for only one week
Alomide®	Lodoxamide	Can produce transient burning but very effective
Cromolyn (generic)	Cromolyn	Often used for long-term usage; difficult to obtain
Steroid drops	Cortisone	Extremely effective *but* when used inappropriately, can cause dangerous complications or side effects; any use should be OK'd by your doctor

junctivitis is abrupt and leads to extremely itchy eyes. It is very uncomfortable for children. Children with vernal conjunctivitis often do not have other allergies, and may be completely free of hay fever or other common allergic symptoms. Because of its seasonal onset, it is thought to be allergic, but we do not know exactly what causes it. The best way to determine if your child has this condition is to have an examination by an allergist or an eye doctor. The doctor will invert the eye lid to look at its underside; where vernal conjunctivitis is involved, the underside of the lid has a characteristic and unmistakable cobblestone appearance. Treatment calls for oral antihistamines, eyedrops, and (very important) avoiding scratching the eyes. Fortunately, most children eventually grow out of this condition by the late teens.

Contact Lenses

A special form of eye irritation is seen in people who wear the newer plastic contact lenses. It is rare in young children (most of whom do not wear contacts), but is found in adolescents and certainly young adults. Children—and adults—who do wear the new plastic contact lenses can develop a condition known as follicular hyperplasia. It results from inappropriate or incomplete cleansing of the contact lens. This may trigger an allergic response resulting in blurring of vision and significant irritation of the eyes. The best treatment for this condition is to avoid the cause—in other words, wear eyeglasses. Although many ophthalmologists allow patients to continue to wear their contacts when this condition develops, persisting with the contact lenses can prove harmful and damaging to the eyes. Also, if you use eye drops be certain that they do not interfere with your contacts. Fewer problems have been reported with the newer disposable contact lenses, but the same cautionary notes described above are still applicable.

Eye Examinations

The eyes are a vital sense organ and remind us of an important additional note. In some schools, eye tests are administered to virtually every child every year, and if the exam is failed, the child is referred to his or her doctor. In other places, the exam may occur once every several years or not at all. Children doing badly in school are often referred to allergists. This happens because of the persistent misconception that obscure, undiagnosed allergies, even in otherwise healthy-appearing children, can impair their ability to learn. Sometimes we find the problem is nothing more than poor vision.

> Sean is an active and seemingly very bright 8-year-old who has great difficulty in reading. School officials thought his reading problem was the result of allergies. It quickly became apparent to his allergist that he suffered from a condition known as dyslexia. Dyslexia, a complex, but not uncommon perceptual problem, is not due to allergies. Sean simply got lost in the mass of students and managed to get by each year without receiving an accurate diagnosis *and* help. Sean was referred to a reading tutor in his district. Over the next several years, he was able to make enormous progress.

Care of the Eyes

As a parent, make it a point to have your child's vision checked periodically; weak or defective eyesight can drastically lower school performance. Reading difficulties, like dyslexia, can be brought out by having your child read aloud to you. If there seems to be trouble recognizing simple words in context, consult with the child's teacher and the school's or district's reading specialist.

There is an old warning that says "never put anything smaller than your elbow in your eye." The eyes are precious, and nothing should be placed in them, medication or otherwise, without help and advice. Since there are numerous medications available for ocular use, there is a tendency for family members to share drugs. We urge you to remember that the treatment for Judy's red eyes may need to be very different than the one for her mother's red eyes.

16

Earache

Earaches in children are usually the result of an infection in the middle ear. They are one of the most frustrating problem of parents and a source of great pain to a child. *Otitis media*, the medical name for the condition, means earache.

Stacey's parents well remember her fourth birthday. She woke up that day cranky and irritable; her parents thought it might be because of excitement in anticipation of the day's activities. The party went badly since Stacey had a series of atypical crying fits and temper tantrums. By evening, the parents sensed that she might be ill. They took her temperature and, finding that it was 101°F, gave her some liquid Tylenol, which brought the fever down and quieted her. At 2:00 the following morning, Stacey awakened, screaming and crying uncontrollably. She complained that her ears hurt. Her temperature was 103°F and she could not be comforted. Her dad, frantic, bundled her up and took her to the local emergency room, where the doctor examined her ears and said that she had a bulging eardrum, characteristic of acute otitis media. Stacey's parents had never heard of otitis media, but they were quick to learn how common chronic infected ears can be. Stacey was given an antibiotic and some medicine for her fever. Within a few hours, she felt better and her temperature quickly returned to normal. Over the next year, though, Stacey had five more of these episodes. Her parents thought an allergy might be responsible and took the child to an allergist. The allergist took a careful history, and quickly concluded that this was all a byproduct of colds and the unique anatomy of children's eustachian tubes and ear canals. No allergy was implicated in her case.

Incidence

As near as we can judge, about one-half of all children have an earache at least once; chronic, recurrent earaches are among the more frequently encountered problems in the pediatrician's office. Boys, obese children, and allergic children (or children of allergic parents) tend to be more susceptible to earaches. The more often a child has a cold, the more the risk of earaches.

Usual Age of Onset

Earache owing to infection is a childhood disease, and is mainly seen in infants, toddlers, and especially preschoolers. It becomes increasingly less prevalent in older age groups, and rarely shows in adolescents or adults. This age-related drop in prevalence of symptoms is a direct result of maturation and the physiological changes that accompany it.

Symptoms

The symptoms of an earache are not directly observable by you, the parent. Indeed, they are likely to turn up in children too young to tell you exactly how they feel. What you observe in the behavior and appearance of the child lets you know of or suspect its presence. An ear infection can make its presence known in a variety of ways:

Acute:
Tugging of the earlobe.
Excruciating pain accompanied by severe distress, crying, and restlessness.
Fever, sometimes quite elevated (103°F+).

Chronic:
Persistent mild, dull earache.
Sense of fullness or stuffiness in the head ("My head feels funny").
"Popping" sensation in the ears, like the one that accompanies rapid changes in elevation.
Low-grade fever.

Temporary or permanent hearing loss is a common and serious aspect of acute or chronic ear infections in children. Indications of hearing loss are subtle and develop almost imperceptibly.

Be alert to the following signs of hearing impairment in your youngsters, especially if there are recurrent bouts of earache.

Inattentiveness, slowness in attending or responding to others, disobedience.
Need for you to speak loudly or to repeat what you have said in order to be understood.
In school-age children, underachievement, withdrawal.

There are also a few physical tipoffs to the possibility of ear infection.

In infants or young children, incessant tugging or clawing at the ear.
Allergic "shiners"—dark shadows under the eyes.
Mouth breathing. This suggests that the nose is chronically stuffed and, possibly, the ear blocked as well. (Mouth breathers often complain of a

bad morning taste in the mouth. This is because the mouth is dried out from the passage of air through it rather than the nose.)

Causes

Earaches result from a structural, anatomical flaw in children. The eustachian tube, a short, slender pipe that connects ear and nose is much smaller in diameter, runs more horizontally, and has a thicker lining of mucous tissue in children than it does in adults. When an upper respiratory infection (colds or flu) hits or nasal allergies (hay fever, perennial allergic rhinitis— *see* Chapter 12) show up, the eustachian tube can become clogged and inflamed. All debris in the tube becomes trapped inside; a bacterial infection then develops in the middle ear and exerts pressure on the eardrum. Pain and the other symptoms described above follow.

The blockage of the immature eustachian tube results most often from viral colds and allergies, generally with a secondary bacterial infection. However, there are other causes as well, including colds, allergies, enlarged adenoids, foreign objects, cleft palate, injuries, and rarely, nasopharyngeal cancer.

When to See the Doctor

Because of the extreme pain and discomfort involved and the distinct threat of hearing impairment that chronic, untreated ear infections present, you should consult your doctor at the first sign of an earache. An untreated earache, if the result of a bacterial infection, can even lead to meningitis and death.

If your child is allergic, any examination of the child in connection with the allergic condition should always include a look into the ears. If the doctor overlooks this important step, offer a gentle reminder to carry it out. ("Wouldn't you like to examine the ears, too?")

First Aid and Home Treatment of Earache

For the child who is susceptible to ear infections, the first and most effective line of treatment is prevention.

Where the earaches are allergy-related (and they will be allergy-related only if allergic symptoms like hay fever or asthma are also present), identify and avoid the agent responsible. (*See* Chapter 6 for information on how to avoid or control airborne allergens.)

Where the earaches are owing to respiratory infections, follow the procedures given in Chapter 5 and 20 to reduce exposure to and to control colds and coughs.

In addition, in infants *avoid* the use of pacifiers, poorly vented nursing bottle nipples, feeding the baby when it is supine, or bottle-propping (for self-feeding), since all of these practices can result in aspiration of fluid into and eventual infection in the middle ear.

You may also want to consider humidifying the sleeping room (*see* Chapter 20 for suggestions about humidifiers) to help keep the respiratory membranes moist and functioning effectively.

Treatment for earache is ordinarily doctor-initiated; folk remedies for it are ineffectual. Where an allergy is responsible, a prescription antihistamine decongestant is usually administered. If bacterial infection is also present, an antibiotic will be prescribed and ordinarily clears up the infection rapidly.

Carefully follow the physician's and pharmacist's instructions about frequency and duration of administration of medications. Neglecting to do this—stopping antibiotics too soon, for example—can result in a quick and stubborn rebound of the infection. Insist on getting information on and be alert to possible side effects from any medications prescribed. If side effects develop, notify your physician at once.

Finally, do not probe or attempt to put anything into the ear. This practice can cause serious damage to the delicate structures in the ear and result in injury and hearing loss.

Long-Term Treatment

If your young child develops acute ear infections several times per year, you should seriously consider having ear tubes implanted. These are plastic inserts that are put in the ears by an ear, nose, and throat specialist. The plastic tubes help drain and ventilate the ear canal, thereby reducing the risk of developing recurrent infections. It is a minor surgical procedure performed on an outpatient basis and often proves extremely helpful. In addition, when the tubes are implanted the physician has the opportunity to remove any fluid or debris that has remained trapped behind the eardrums. This removal of fluid acts to prevent further infection or even hearing loss.

Ear tubes do carry some disadvantages you ought to know about. In very young children, they have a tendency to fall out. This is troublesome, although essentially harmless. Children with air tube implants must either use earplugs or exercise extreme care to avoid getting water into their ears while bathing. Swimming or showering should be avoided.

Ear tubes are not for everyone and work best for younger children with recurrent problems that are not rapidly responsive to antibiotics. We should also note that the overall effectiveness of ear tubes has been questioned. In our experience, they work best for young children (less than six years old) who have more than four ear infections per year. Moreover, if your child responds rapidly to antibiotics (within 24 hours), the ear tubes are probably not needed.

Complications of Earaches

Hearing loss, temporary or permanent, is a common companion of ear infections.

Holly is an 11 year-old who is an excellent reader, but seems not to follow verbal directions well. Although she is a pleasant and attractive youngster, she is often seen playing alone, in and out of school. She was referred to an allergist because her school performance seemed far below her potential as evidenced by test scores. As part of the exam, the allergist looked in her ears. The eardrums appeared normal, but her tympanogram was abnormal. (A tympanogram is a test that measures the ability of the eardrum to retract.) The doctor wondered whether she had a gluey ear from chronic untreated ear infections, so he referred her to an audiologist who found that Holly had a minor, but significant hearing deficit. The audiologist helped her enormously with a hearing aid. Holly's immediate reaction, when the device was installed, was to ask "Why is everybody shouting?" Holly quickly adapted to it, and although her hearing is not completely normal, her parents and teachers are amazed at how much her school performance and her social relationships have improved.

You can crudely assess the possibility of a hearing loss in your child by using a watch—one that ticks, of course. In a quiet room with the child seated and facing away from you, move the watch toward the child's ear until ticking is heard; note the distance from watch to ear. Then put the watch close to the ear where the child reports hearing it and move it away to the point where it becomes inaudible. Note the distance. Repeat for the other ear. Compare distances with someone who has not experienced ear troubles—another child, perhaps, or your spouse. If the distances are substantially lower for the child, tell your doctor, who may order more sophisticated tests by a hearing specialist.

Ear Allergies

Middle ear infections, although they can be caused by allergies, are not allergies as such, and the medications prescribed for treatment of middle ear infections are not aimed at and have no effect on them. However, topical antibiotics put into the ear for treatment of certain local infections—swimmer's itch in particular—can cause a contact allergy, either from the antibiotic or the paste that serves as its vehicle. Your child may be given a topical antibiotic for a superficial ear infection; the ear seems to get better. Then, the skin in the ear canal gets red and the infection seems to grow much worse. Actually, the ear infection is not involved, but an allergic reaction to the antibiotic or its base has set in. If this should happen, discontinue the medication at once, and check with your doctor.

Traveling with an Earache

The eustachian tube is very important in exchanging air between the nose and the ear. If the middle ear begins to become clogged, a fair amount of pain can result. In fact, keeping the eustachian tube open is extremely important. Generally, every time you yawn, chew, or swallow, the tubes open and air is allowed to go through the middle ear. Virtually anyone who has been in an airplane has experienced the popping sensation that occurs as the plane descends to lower altitudes. This is owing to the exchange of air between the outside and inside of the ear. In some people, especially children, with clogged eustachian tubes, this exchange of air may not occur and intense pain results. The pain can be associated with a temporary loss of hearing and ear infections. Thus, if your child is going to ride in an airplane or travel to the mountains, make sure the ears are clear. If your children are susceptible to ear infections, it would not hurt to give them an over-the-counter antihistamine-decongestant before the trip. In fact, one of the very few indications for use of an intranasal decongestant, like Afrin, is prior to a trip, if your child is old enough to be treated with such a medicine. This treatment, although it is only temporary, may also help open the ear canal.

> Every time Nikki and her family traveled from her home in California's central valley to the family summer home in the High Sierras, her daughter developed a severe earache, which kept her uncomfortable for several days. It always ruined the family vacation. Finally after many such episodes, Nikki made the connection between her daughter's ears and high altitude. She saw her doctor, who found that Nikki's daughter had a chronic accumulation of fluid in her middle ear. Nikki was totally unaware that her daughter had been having this problem. Her daughter was treated with antibiotics and antihistamine decongestants, and the condition cleared up very rapidly. Afterward, until her daughter reached age 8, Nikki routinely gave her a decongestant before they went up to the mountains. She quickly found that it was only the change in altitude, rather than the altitude itself, that was a problem.

Tonsillectomies and Adenoidectomies

Adenoids and tonsils are soft-tissue lymph nodes in the nasal airways. In some children, when enlarged, these structures can cause significant obstruction of the airway and/or constriction of the eustachian tube. When it appears clear beyond doubt that they are implicated in respiratory problems or recurrent ear infections, their surgical removal may be advisable. However, the old practice of routinely taking out tonsils and adenoids has been abandoned as useless, if not actually harmful. For some children—those with a cleft palate or who have other speaking problems or handicaps—tonsillectomies or adenoidectomies may seriously impair speech and should be avoided if at all possible.

17

Plant (Poison Oak or Ivy) and Other Causes of Contact Dermatitis

Allergic and Irritant Contact Dermatitis

Allergic contact dermatitis is an inflammation of the skin characterized by redness and the formation of vesicles; vesicles are similar to blisters. Allergic contact dermatitis occurs after exposure to a wide variety of substances—many of which are also capable of causing nonallergic irritation. This irritant reaction appears following injury to cells as a result of direct contact with the offending substance; the allergic response develops after repeated contacts with a sensitizer, which eventually provokes an immune inflammatory side reaction in the body. In practice, it is often difficult to distinguish allergic from irritant contact dermatitis. Table 20 lists ways in which they differ.

Contact dermatitis can be expressed in a variety of ways, and can be either allergic or nonallergic (irritant) in origin. It is a generic term applied to a broad group of skin irritations, rashes, or eruptions arising from contact with a substance responsible for producing symptoms by a susceptible person. Certainly the most notorious triggers of contact dermatitis are members of the Rhus group of plants, especially poison oak, poison ivy, and poison sumac. Upward of 50% of Americans are sensitive to these plants.

Eddie, 8 years old, takes being a Cub Scout seriously and listens intently to everything the pack's Den Mother says. On Arbor Day the youngsters go on a field trip to a Nature Center, where they see several species of birds, are told about the various forms of plant and animal life in the Center, and are permitted to explore on their own while the parents prepare a picnic for the boys. "Be back here in 30 minutes for lunch" they are told. Eddie returns right on time carrying a plant. "Is this the three-leafed one you told us to watch out for?"

Table 20
Types of Contact Dermititis

Symptom	Irritant	Allergic
Time to onset after exposure	Rapid—usually within a few hours	Leisurely—from 1 day to as long as a week
Type of reaction	Red, scaling, and with blisters; painful	Red with small pimples; itchy
Extent or distribution	Confined to area of exposure	May spread widely

he asked the leader innocently. "It sure is, Eddie," the leader said. "Please put it over there on the ground. Now why don't you come with me while we wash you up. The rest of you go over and look at what Eddie has found. Look but don't touch, OK? That is poison oak and we are going to take Eddie to the restroom and have him wash so he will not get a rash from picking it." This was an astute move on her part, exactly right, but no use. Eddie took the beginnings of a nice case of poison oak home with him.

Incidence

Almost any substance can cause a skin rash in a susceptible person and almost everyone, at some time or another, touches something that does provoke a reaction.

Nobody accurately knows the number of individuals suffering from allergic contact dermatitis. We do know that with the growing intrusion of chemicals into all aspects of contemporary life, the complaint will become more prevalent.

Usual Age of Onset

Rashes resulting from contact with irritants can occur at any age. Children are especially susceptible to certain irritants—notably feces and urine in diapers and certain chemicals commonly found in and around the house—and they may show symptoms as early as the first few weeks or even days of life. Because allergic reactions usually develop only after repeated exposure over a period of time, dermatitis in infants or very young children is likely to be the irritant type.

Symptoms

Acute contact dermatitis is characterized by itching (often so severe as to be almost unbearable), reddening of the skin, and the eruption of patches of blisters where the irritant has touched the skin. The itching may be accompanied by scaling and crusting if the dermatitis persists or

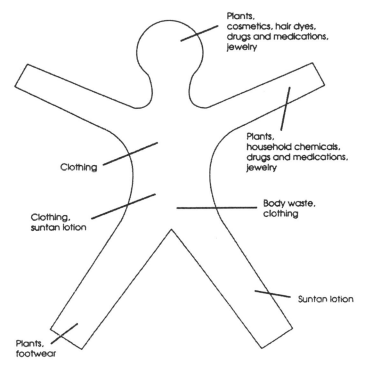

Fig. 7. Common sites of contact dermatitis.

becomes chronic; the skin often thickens, and becomes leathery and striated in the affected areas.

Causes

If your child turns up with contact dermatitis, the chances are therefore fairly good that one of the following agents is responsible:

Body wastes: urine, feces;

Plants: poison oak, ivy, or sumac;

Household chemicals: detergents, polishes, waxes, insecticides, disinfectants;

Drugs and medications: skin medications for cuts, scratches, insect bites, sunburn; topical antihistamines; drugs with names ending in "caine" like benzocaine; topical antibiotics, especially penicillin, neomycin;

Cosmetics: toilet soaps, perfumed oils and lotions, lipstick, nail polish, hair dyes;

Clothing and footwear: wool; chemicals applied to garments to retard flame or for sizing; chemicals used in processing or curing leather or rubber footwear.

Table 21

First Aid and Home Treatment for Common Allergic Skin Disorders

Complaint and symptoms	Common causes	Treatment
Plant dermatitis (Red rash and small blisters; severe itching)	Contact with poison ivy, oak, sumac	1. Learn to identify the plants accurately to avoid them. 2. Avoid contact with pets (dogs especially) that roam in areas where the plants grow 3. If exposed, flush the site of contact immediately with cold water 4. If a reaction occurs, apply steroid creams or ointments like Cortaid 5. If symptoms are severe and widespread, see a physician for prescription of oral steroid
Diaper dermatitis (Hives and blister-like pimples in the area covered by the diaper; body folds or creases often less involved)	Overlong contact with feces or urine; soap or detergents remaining in diapers	1. Change diapers frequently 2. Wash diapers carefully and rinse thoroughly 3. Clean skin with mild soap and water; rinse well; if irritation is severe, substitute olive or mineral oil for soap 4. *Do not* use plastic diaper covers (plastic-coated disposable diapers, which keep urine away from the skin, are acceptable) 5. Apply zinc oxide ointment to affected area 6. If above steps prove ineffectual, consult a physician
Foot dermatitis (Red, thickened, scaly, itchy sores)	Chemicals or other substances used in manufacture of shoes (patch test required for accurate diagnosis)	1. Wear cotton or other non-reactive socks 2. If necessary, purchase made-to-order, allergy-free footwear 3. Apply steroid ointment several times daily; bandage with airtight dressing at night.
Clothing dermatitis (Red rash and blister-like pimples where clothing in contact with skin)	Wool clothing, overly tight clothing; soaps or detergents remaining in garments; flame-retardant sleepwear	1. Avoid wearing offending fabric 2. Rinse clothes carefully after washing 3. If necessary, apply salves or steroid creams or ointments

144

(Continued)

Table 21 (*Continued*)

Complaint and symptoms	Common causes	Treatment
Soap and detergent dermatitis (rashing and scaling of skin)	Too frequent or too prolonged bathing; excessive use of bubble bath	1. Bathe less often 2. Eliminate bubble bath 3. Use salves or emollients to counteract skin dryness
Cosmetic and medication dermatitis (rashing, eruption, scaling of skin)	Lipsticks, powders, nail polish, hair dye; names of products or substances ending in "caine" (surfocaine, benzocaine); anti-itch, sunburn, and poison oak remedies; antihistamine and antibiotic ointments and their preservatives (patch test frequently necessary because of number of possible offenders)	1. Avoid use or contact with substance responsible 2. Apply steroid salves or ointments

145

The list above is not meant to be complete; it simply identifies some of the more common causes of contact dermatitis.

First Aid and Home Treatment of Contact Dermatitis

Effective treatment of your child's contact dermatitis depends on your carrying out two steps successfully. They are: (1) identifying and then avoiding the cause of the reaction and (2) looking after the sores or lesions appropriately.

The cause of the reaction can usually be inferred by carefully reviewing the activities or experiences that your child has had recently—especially new or different ones—and trying to link them to the place or places on the body where the lesions have appeared. Figure 7 indicates the places on your child's body where various forms of contact dermatitis are likely to turn up initially. Table 21 lists the most common allergic skin disorders, their causes, and how to treat them.

Long-Term Treatment

If you pin down the cause of your child's dermatitis accurately, prevent further contact with it, *and* follow the appropriate treatment spelled out in Table 21 faithfully, the problem should be resolved. However, you should see your doctor if:

Infection is present.

The rash, after a few days' treatment, fails to improve or gets worse; or you cannot establish the cause when the dermatitis is caused by medications or chemicals, the offending agent may be obscure and difficult to identify; in these cases, accurate diagnosis calls for a patch test, which your doctor will have to carry out.

Special Hints

If the cause is correctly identified and the proper treatment is followed, symptoms should clear within a week or two and should not return unless avoidance procedures break down. Normally contact dermatitis, if treated promptly and effectively, will not cause any permanent damage or disfigurement.

Part Four

General Health Problems: Their Special Importance In Children With Allergies

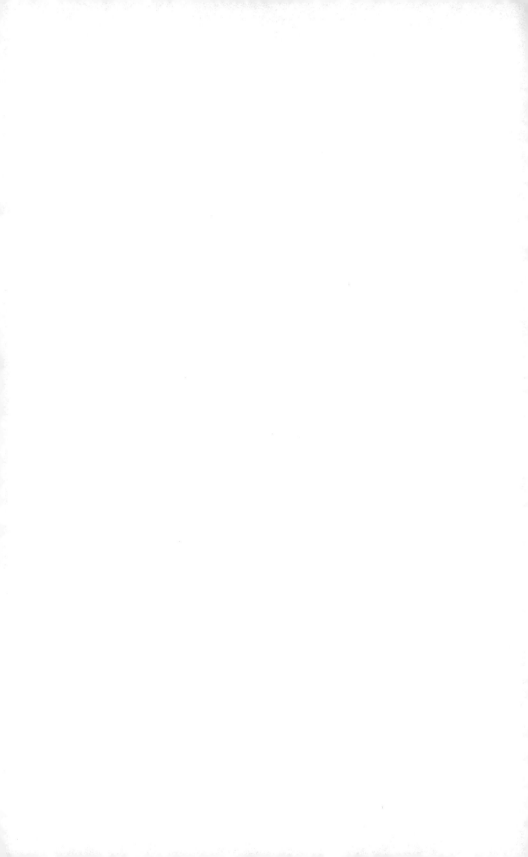

18

Headache

Incidence

Headaches are relatively uncommon in childhood. When they do occur, they should be taken seriously because they are often associated with special circumstances that have significant health implications, particularly for allergic children.

Usual Age of Onset

Headaches can occur at any age. Because their most frequent cause is stress growing out of everyday life, they are much more prevalent in adults.

Symptoms

Children's headaches can be roughly identified according to their perceived location and the nature of the pain itself (*see* Table 22).

When a child complains that his or her head hurts: First, determine, if you can, whether the headache is the result of a blow or injury. ("Tell me what happened.") If a trauma is responsible and it appears serious or if the pain persists for more than a short period of time, call or see your doctor. Second, have the child indicate the location of the pain ("Where does it hurt?") and its nature. ("Does it hurt all the time?" "Does it come and go?"). These steps are important in identifying the likely cause and deciding what to do about treatment.

Causes

In children, the major cause of headache is *fever*—especially a temperature over 103°F (40°C). The fever may be accompanied by nausea and vomiting. Note that fever is a sign or symptom, not a disease in itself. *See* Chapter 19 for more about fever.

Jay came home from school feeling a bit tired. His babysitter was a little surprised that Jay went to the couch and quickly fell asleep. Usually the first thing he did was to turn on the television and watch cartoons. She decided to

Table 22
Type of Pain, Usual Location, and Common Causes of Chronic Headache

	USUAL LOCATION			
Type of Pain	Both sides of head	One side of head	Behind the eye	Above or below eye
Steady ache	Stress or tension			
Intense, throbbing		Migraine[a]		
Piercing, burning			Vascular	
Pressure-like				Sinus
Causes	Stress; emotional problems; jaw-clenching; tooth grinding	Spasms or inflammation of blood vessels; stress	Dietary factors; see Table 23	Sinus infection; congestion of sinuses owing to allergy

[a]Migraine, an extremely complicated condition, has special characteristics. Most migraine sufferers, even before the pain starts, know that it is coming. These preliminary warning symptoms (called the "aura") can include feelings of weakness, light-headedness, severe nausea, sweatiness or clamminess, dizziness, tremor, extreme sensitivity to sound and light, and cold hands and feet. A child with what appears to be migraine should see a neurologist for a firm diagnosis and to have appropriate treatment prescribed.

wake him up after about an hour and ask if he was ill. When aroused he said that he had a very bad headache. He looked flushed, so she took his temperature and found it to be 103°F. Jay did not realize he had a fever, but shortly after the babysitter took his temperature, he began to vomit. She gave him some Tylenol; his temperature dropped within an hour, and his headache disappeared.

Headaches may also result from foods or other substances that contain chemicals called vasoactive amines. Vasoactive amines cause the blood vessels in the brain to constrict and dilate, and this process produces vascular headache. Table 23 lists foods containing headache-causing vasoactive amines.

In addition, some children may be made violently ill by certain foods that induce nausea, vomiting, or severe diarrhea. This acute physiological stress can also cause dilation of blood vessels and a headache.

A few children will show the acute pain and other symptoms associated with migraine headaches. Migraine is also vascular; it runs in families; it is not the result of allergies; and because of its severity and the possibility that the symptoms can be produced by an imposter, if you suspect that your child

Table 23
Foods Containing Vasoactive Amines

I.	Chocolate, cocoa, fava beans
2.	All ripened cheeses
3.	Avocados
4.	Bananas
5.	Canned figs
6.	Fermented sausage (i.e., bologna, salami, pepperoni, aged beef, hot dogs)
7.	Red wine, sherry
8.	Beer
9.	Chicken livers
I0.	Pickled herring
II.	Anchovies
I2.	Dried fish
I3.	Yeast extracts (breads and candy)

has migraine, you should arrange for a consultation with a neurologist as soon as possible. Moreover, there are many new treatments for migraine headache, and no one should suffer needlessly.

Elizabeth has had headaches since she was 4 years of age. She knows exactly when they will begin. About an hour before the headache she begins to develop a sense of flushing throughout her body. Then, within minutes, ordinary light seems to hurt her eyes. (This pain from light is called photophobia.) Within 15 minutes thereafter, the headache begins. It is an incredibly pounding headache that makes her weak all over, unable to do anything more than lie down in bed. It usually lasts between 4 and 12 hours and only gets better when she takes the special migraine medicine her neurologist prescribed.

Psychological stress—extreme anxiety, tension, conflict—can also produce headache, although these so-called tension headaches are extremely uncommon in children.

Malcolm is considered a brilliant student; he has made virtually straight A's all of his life. He is anxiously awaiting taking his college entrance exams and has been studying very hard for them. It is quite common for Malcolm to get headaches. Most often the headaches develop from lack of sleep. Recently, the headaches have been coming on virtually every morning before he goes to school. His mother thinks he is not eating enough and has been trying to feed him more. The result has been that he is now becoming obese. Malcolm has confided to his friends that his parents have an obsession about his making high grades and he worries constantly that he will fail.

Withdrawal from caffeine or caffeine-like substances also causes dilation of blood vessels and a sharp, throbbing headache. Although not often encountered in children, it sometimes occurs a few hours after the child consumes significant amounts of caffeine, especially in soft drinks like cola. It is also seen fairly often in asthmatic children who are taking theophylline to control their wheezing.

Hard physical exertion—running, jumping, bouts of sneezing, coughing, and so forth—is occasionally associated with the sudden onset of, usually, short-lived headaches. Also ingesting very cold food or drink (ice cream, chilled soda) can cause a transient headache around the temples.

First Aid and Home Treatment of Headaches

Figure 8 traces the steps to follow in treating your child's headache.

Special Hints or Warnings

Aspirin: When a headache hits, most older people think immediately of taking an aspirin. For a child—or for an allergic person of any age—this can be dangerous. *Never, for any reason, administer aspirin to a child.* Use acetaminophin (Tylenol) or a generic brand instead. There are two reasons for this stern advice: (1) Aspirin is associated with Reye's syndrome, an almost always fatal disease in children. It often develops after the use of aspirin to control fever brought on by flu or chicken pox. (2) Aspirin can have severe effects on people with allergies. It can trigger asthma or make it worse, sometimes causing status asthmaticus and hospitalization.

Carl developed asthma following an upper respiratory infection at age three. For the next several years, his asthma always got worse whenever he got a cold. The cold would start in his nose and then move down in his chest. He saw a variety of doctors for this, but no one seemed to help him as much as his family would have liked. He took a whole variety of asthma medications for it, seemingly doing everything he was supposed to. Finally, his pediatrician asked his mom whether Carl ever gets aspirin for fever. She said no, absolutely not. She had been told many times that children with asthma should not be given aspirin. She said she only uses Anacin. "Anacin!" the doctor cried. Anacin contains aspirin!!"

In fact, aspirin is found in over 100 over-the-counter products for colds, congestion, some sleeping pills, and others. Table 24 names medications, including cold "remedies," that contain aspirin. *Avoid these scrupulously!*

"Food" Headaches

Do not fall for the claim that headaches are the result of some complex, rare, mysterious reaction to foods. Headache can result from the presence of certain vasoactive amines in the foods named in Table 23. Children who develop headaches without fever should be asked exactly what they have eaten that day and their inventory checked against the table. If matches occur, eliminate the suspected offender, and keep track to see if the headache goes away.

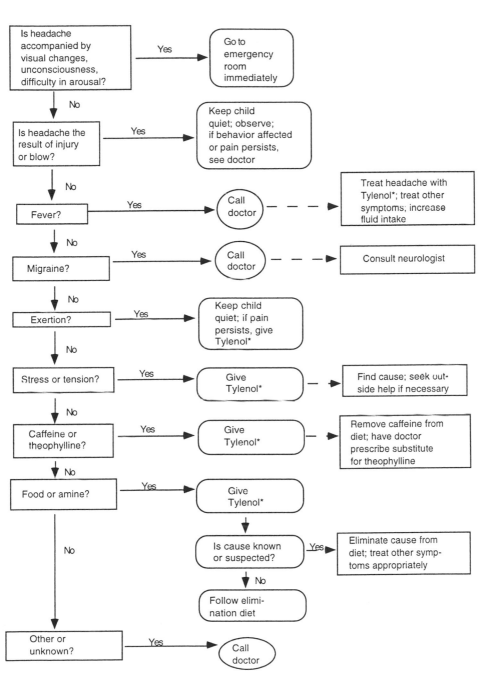

See page 152 for explanation of Tylenol recommendation.

Fig. 8.

Table 22
Common Medicines that Contain Asprin

A.P.C.	Cold Tablets	Norgesic
Acedyne Wafer	Coralsone	Orphenadrine
Aluprin	Coricidin	P-A-C Compound
Aminodyne Compound	Dasikon	Pain Reliever-E
Anacin	Dasin	Phencoid
Analgesic Compound	Docaphen	Phenergan Compound
Analgestine Forte	Dolene Compound-65	Phenetron Compound
Analgets Water	Dolor Plus	Pirseal
Anaphen	Dovacet	Poxy Compound-65
Andquan	Doverin	Presalin
Anexsia-D	Dovosal	Progesic Compound-65
Anodynos-DHC	Drinophen	Propoxyphene Compound
Antrin	Dristan	Proxene Compound
Apac	Duradyne	Pyrroxate
Apacomp	Duragesic	Quiet World
Aphonals	Dynosal	Repro Compound-65
Arthritis Pain Formula	Ecotrin	Rhinate
As-Ca-Phen	Emagrin Forte	Rhinex
Ascriptin	Empirin Analgesic	Rid-A-Col
Aspergum	Emprazil	Roxaxisal
Asphac-G	Equagesic	Ru-Lor
Aspir-I0	Esemgesic	Sal-Fayne
Aspirbar	Ex Apap	Salagen
Aspirin	Excedrin	Saleto
Aspirin Buffered	Febro-Bar	Salocol
Atokas	Fidgesic	Salphenine
Axotal	Fiorinal	Sine-Off
B-A	Fizrin	Sine-Aid Sinus Headache Tablets
Bayer	Gelcoid	SK-65 Compound
B-A	I-PAC	St. Joseph Aspirin
Bayer Aspirin	ICN 65 Compound	St. Joseph Aspirin for Children
Bayer Children's Chewable Aspirin	Idenal	Stanback Analgesic
Bayer Timed-Release Aspirin	Isobutal	Steradrin
Bexophene	Isollyl	Supac
Buff-A	Lanaba	Synalgos
Buffadyne-Lemmon	Lanorinal	Synalgos-DC
Bufferin	Liqualgine	Talwin Compound
Buffex	Marflex Plus	Ten-Shun
Buffinol	Margesic Compound 65	Trigesic
Butalbital Compound	Marnal	Valacet
Butalbital with A.P.C.	Measurin	Valdeine
Cafacetin	Mepro Compound	Valesin
Capron	Meprogesic	Valobar
Carbrogesic	Methocarbamol with Aspirin	Valophen
Christodyne DHC	Micrainin	Vanquish
Cirin	Midol	Vasogesic
Citroval	Momentum	Viromed
Codasa 30 mg	Nilain	Zactirin

Sherry occasionally gets headaches that always seem to occur about an hour or two after eating cheese. Because she is convinced that this is from an allergy to foods, her mother took her to the doctor to discuss it. Her doctor knows that fresh cheese is rich in vasoactive amines, that Sherry is more sensitive to vasoactive amines than other people, and probably has a headache secondary to this. He had Sherry write down everything she ate over a 2-week period, and he also had her record the times of the day when she developed a headache. Sherry realized even before she went back to her doctor that she developed a headache every time she ate fresh cheese.

Fortunately, most of us never develop a vasoactive amine headache. To the minority who do, however, missing the diagnosis of the trigger may forebode a life of suffering.

19

Fever

Incidence

Children of any age can and most, at some point, do develop fever. It can appear quickly and, in infants and children, often rises to alarmingly high levels, although children tolerate temperature extremes more readily than adolescents or adults.

Symptoms

A fever is simply an above-normal body temperature. A normal temperature (taken orally) is defined as 98.6°F or 36.9°C. In practice, the healthy individual's temperature will show slight variations from the normal from one day to another and according to the time of day and the type of activity being pursued. Some individuals may have a personal "normal," which is slightly higher or lower than the average 98.6°F.

Causes

Fever is a symptom provoked by any of literally hundreds of causes. Infections, colds in particular, are the most common causes of fever. A fever is an indication that something is wrong. It should not be left unattended or trifled with. A high, untreated fever can have devasting consequenes, including seizures. For some reason, very young children have higher fevers than adults.

Allergies *do not* induce fever. "Hay fever," the popular term for allergic rhinitis, has no effect on body temperature. The term "hay fever", like so many others in medicine, persists in widespread use, although it is incorrect and misleading.

Even though fever is not the result of allergies, children with allergies may be severely affected by fever because fever accelerates the metabolic rate. Heartbeat and respiratory rate speed up, and these developments can trigger or intensify some allergic conditions—eczema and asthma in particular. Because of this, detecting the presence of even a slight fever and returning the body temperature of allergic children to normal during infections—colds especially—are extremely important. For example, breathing rapidly, whether from a fever or from exercise, can make asthma worse.

First Aid and Home Treatment of Fever

Treatment of fever has several steps:

1. Measure the temperature accurately, and record the value, time, and date. See Table 25 for procedures to follow in taking a temperature correctly.
2. Determine the cause of the fever: Never treat a fever until you are sure what you are treating! If the condition responsible is not immediately apparent and unmistakable, see the doctor. Reasons for this caution are that the presence of the fever often helps the doctor to diagnose what is happening. Treating it beforehand may temporarily make the child feel better while the underlying cause is smoldering and getting worse. (A child with acute abdominal pain and fever, for instance, can feel better with Tylenol, but if the cause of the fever is appendicitis, appropriate treatment may be delayed with potentially grave consequences.)
3. Treat the fever: Treatment of fever in children consists of administering acetaminophen and applying other measures, like sponge baths, which will lower the surface temperature of the body. The appropriate dosage of acetaminophen is determined by age. Table 26 gives dosages according to age. Do not give aspirin to children.
4. Do not treat fever in children with aspirin in any form: As noted in the preceding chapter, treating fevers with aspirin has been linked with Reye's Syndrome, an often fatal disease in children.

Aspirin also triggers or intensifies certain allergic reactions, especially asthma, and should not be used by a child or adult who has them. It can also cause bleeding and gastric ulcers.

June has had recurrent colds and infections throughout her childhood. She does not have allergies. Her mother remembers the old days when aspirin was used routinely for fever. No one ever told her that aspirin can induce ulcers. June has been under a fair amount of stress; she has been absent so much during the school year that her work is suffering. She has a temperature of 101°F, and her mother has been giving her two aspirin every 4 to 6 hours during the daytime. June has been complaining that her stomach has been bothering her and her stools have been turning black and tarry. Her mother thought it might be from the multiple vitamins containing iron. At 2:00 in the morning, June woke up, felt extremely sick, and began to vomit blood. She was rushed to the hospital and diagnosed as having an aspirin-induced ulcer.

Table 25
How to Take a Temperature

When using a mercury thermometer:
1. Store the thermometer in its case. (Left loose on the shelf, they invariably fall and break; a broken thermometer, even if the mercury column is unaffected, is dangerous.)
2.* Before use, dip thermometer in ethyl alcohol to guard against reinfection from prior illnesses.
3.** Shake thermometer to drive mercury to base of shaft, near bulb. Check to see that it is down.
4. Insert thermometer. (Temperature may be taken rectally—if proper type of thermometer is used; usually preferable in infants or children 4 to 6 years old.) In case of rectal administration, lubricate with petroleum jelly; do not force; keep child under close surveillance at all times; in oral administration, place bulb under tongue; keep mouth closed, lips encircling thermometer; caution child against biting or moving thermometer.)
5. Leave thermometer in place for *at least* 3 minutes.
6. Remove thermometer. Read result. Write down date, time, and reading. (This information may be useful for your doctor.)
7.* Clean thermometer with cotton, dip in alcohol, shake down, and return to case.

*In steps 2 and 7, swab with alcohol-soaked cotton before and after use.
**When using an electronic or digital thermometer step 3 is not necessary.

Table 26
Dose of Acetominophen to be Administered in Fever

Age in years	Dose^a
Less than 2	50 mg
2–6	70 mg
6–12	150 mg
Over 12	375 mg

^{a}Can be repeated in 20 to 30 minutes if no response. Read directions and bottle labels carefully for specific doses.

5. Increase fluid intake: More fluid is needed during a fever. Use water or apple juice, but not milk. Milk may produce nausea and vomiting.

Complications

Fever, as mentioned above, can provoke or intensify eczema and asthma. Monitor the temperature of your asthma or eczema-prone child regularly, and treat even a slight fever promptly. (Eczema symptoms grow worse with fever; fever also speeds up breathing, which can lead to hyperventilation and asthmatic wheezing.)

Febrile seizures—seizures that resemble acute epilepsy—sometimes happen in children with high fevers. Children subject to this frightening condition should be watched closely and vigorously treated at the first sign of temperature elevation. This aggressive, preventive posture will usually ward off seizures.

20

Coughs and Colds

Incidence

Coughing is one of the most frequent problems in children. Most children will have several colds or coughs per year; pharmacy shelves are loaded with over-the-counter cough remedies, many of them aimed at children.

Usual Age of Onset

Children can turn up with a cough at any age; for allergic children and their parents, colds and coughs take on special significance and need to be watched closely and treated aggressively. The cold/cough-allergy connection is twofold; colds or other respiratory infections are the most common trigger of asthma in children, and a cough is sometimes the only sign of the presence of asthma.

Symptoms

Coughs can take any of several forms and show up at particular times. A cough can be *dry* or *wet*. (A wet cough is one that sounds like it is bringing up phlegm or mucus.) It can be a hoarse croupy cough accompanied by noisy, raspy breathing in infants and young children; it can be around-the-clock or only at night (nocturnal) or it can be the deep, wracking and unique sound of whooping cough, a dangerous, but fortunately uncommon childhood disease.

Causes

The cough, much like fever or headache, is actually a sign that something is wrong. It may be a reaction to a trivial, everyday infection like a cold or flu, or it may be caused by a serious underlying disease like bronchitis, pneumonia, or whooping cough (pertussis), which is brought on by an infection by the Bordetella pertussis bacterium. Whooping cough has special implications for allergic children, and these are discussed under the *Complications* heading later in this chapter.

A chronic cough can also be the result of a foreign object caught in the lung—peanuts, M&M's, other food particles, pencil erasers, paper clips, pieces of toys, and so on.

First Aid and Home Treatment of Coughs and Colds

A cough in a child is almost always self-limiting, moderating and going away by itself after a brief period of time. Steps in treatment of a cough are given in Fig. 9.

When Paula picks up her four-year-old daughter Mary from preschool on Wednesday, she notices that the child is a bit flushed and somewhat cross. When they get home, Paula takes the child's temperature and finds it to be 100.5°F. Mary also begins complaining that her throat hurts. Paula, who knows that many of the children in Mary's room have been troubled by these same symptoms, immediately increases Mary's fluid intake and treats the fever with acetaminophen. By the next morning the symptoms have grown more pronounced; although the fever has dropped a bit, Mary now has a cough and a runny nose. Paula keeps her out of school that day, has her stay inside, continues treating the fever keeps the level of fluid consumption high, and tries to keep her amused without too much success; Mary would rather be at school with her friends. During the day, the cough becomes more pronounced and productive—Mary starts bringing up phlegm—so Paula is fairly confident that this is a simple cold. She keeps Mary out of school over the weekend. By Monday, the symptoms are mainly gone, and Mary is able to return to school without being actively infectious.

The following are other treatment steps.

Humidifiers

It sometimes helps, especially in croupy coughs, to increase the humidity of the bedroom. This can be done by using a vaporizer. Vaporizers can be purchased inexpensively from your local pharmacy. We recommend that the vaporizer you use, to reduce danger of fire and burns, be the type that produces room temperature vapor. It is also important to clean the vaporizer thoroughly with diluted vinegar (including the container and the vaporizing mechanism) during use and before storing it; otherwise, it can become contaminated with mold or other allergens, and put them in the air to aggravate coughs and trigger other symptoms in asthmatics and hay fever sufferers.

Over-the-Counter Cold and Cough Medications

Over-the-counter medications come in a bewildering variety of brand names and forms—liquids, pills, capsules, lozenges. There are two main types of cough medication—suppressants and expectorants.

Cough suppressants are supposed to eliminate the cough. To do this, they rely on a substance called dextromethorphan, but its concentration in

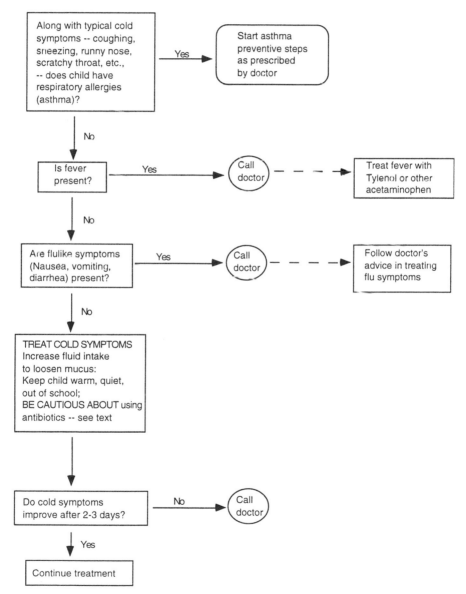

Fig. 9. First aid and home treatment for coughs and colds.

children's over-the-counter cough remedies is too small to be effective. Having the youngster sip clear, warm fruit juices or a mild herb tea with honey can be as effective as the drugstore remedies.

Cough lozenges or drops that are supposed to ease coughing are little more than candy flavored with eucalyptus or horehound to give it a medicinal taste. You can get the same mouth and throat-moistening effect from fruit Life-Savers.

There are effective cough suppressants, but they can only be obtained by prescription. These medications are potent, carry heavy side effects, and are not routinely recommended for children.

Cough expectorants are supposed to act to lubricate and help get rid of the mucus and other material accompanying a cold or respiratory infection. Although the idea is fine in principle, expectorants are not especially effective. A sharp increase in fluid intake will usually accomplish as much at considerably less cost. By "sharp increase" we mean at least double or triple the normal daily intake of (preferably) warm liquids.

Note that some expectorants contain an antihistamine and may have an alcohol base as well. These formulations can have the effect of causing drowsiness or sleepiness, which, in asthmatic children, can impair breathing efficiency and trigger a severe bout of asthma. The antihistamines may also dry out the nose and eustachian tube and bring on earache (otitis media) or severe and stubborn nasal symptoms in susceptible children.

Complications

Whooping cough is a serious, sometimes fatal disease of childhood that was once widely prevalent; mortality rates of as high as 50% from it have been recorded. Children who contract this disease develop a severe cough often associated with a deep breath or "whoop" just before the cough—hence its name. In instances where it proves fatal, the cough becomes nonstop, preventing the child from taking in any air and, in effect, suffocating.

There is a preventive vaccine for whooping cough as well as an effective antibiotic treatment. We believe that every normal child should complete the whooping cough immunization series; however, the whooping cough vaccine carries special, serious implications for allergic children.

Our reasons for concern have to do with some unusual properties of the whooping cough vaccine. It has been shown, in animals, to be an adjuvant, that is, in addition to conferring immunity to Bordetella pertussis, it is capable of inducing high levels of IgE. A high level of IgE in humans can make allergies worse.

Because of this adjuvant property, we recommend that children with moderate to severe allergies and a family history of allergies *as well as* all children with asthma *not* receive whooping cough vaccine. (*See* Chapter 24 for recommendations on vaccination.)

Other allergic children should *not* be vaccinated when they have a cold or other respiratory infection or at times when pollen counts are high.

We recommend that you talk over this problem, if it applies to your child, with your pediatrician or family practitioner. If the doctor seems unaware of the whooping cough vaccine-IgE link, have him or her discuss it with an allergist before making a decision.

Special Hints

Nocturnal cough, a cough that occurs at night with no other symptoms, may be the first and sometimes the only sign of asthma. You, the parent, may resort to treating this annoying sort of cough with any of hundreds of over-the-counter cough medications—usually with no success. The only effective treatment will be one that addresses the underlying asthma.

For children with a nocturnal, asthma-caused cough, we recommend treatment at bedtime with asthma medication as prescribed by your pediatrician or family practitioner. Usually this preventive treatment will make the cough go away. Since the mildest form of asthma is ordinarily implicated in nocturnal cough, it usually vanishes as the child grows older—often by the age of six years or so—and the respiratory airways enlarge.

21

Other Allergic and Pseudo-Allergic Complaints

Allergies catch more than their fair share of the blame when it comes to illness in children. Too many people—physicians among them—wrongly conclude that any condition that resists diagnosis has to be allergic in origin. As a result, allergy has become a catchall diagnosis for a wide variety of baffling conditions, and a steady parade of men, women, and children complaining of a myriad of vague, mysterious symptoms turn up at the allergist's office. This tendency to turn allergy into the Ellis Island of diseases has been abetted by a parallel development—with the accelerating degradation and invasion of the environment by substances that provoke symptoms—allergic and hypersensitivity reactions—that have not previously been encountered.

There are a variety of problems we run into in everyday life as we face daily stresses, and the extent of their impact is not clearly known. Perhaps in the 21st century, we will come to know more about the causes and management of conditions like stress, headaches, depression, agitation, fatigue, hyperactivity, inability to concentrate, and the like. For now, though, these are simply words that strive to describe how one feels—and not at all precisely at that. The sections that follow discuss some of these common syndromes and what we know about them.

Allergic Fatigue or Allergic Tension-Fatigue Syndrome

This syndrome was first described nearly 30 years ago as extreme fatigue often associated with agitation or hyperactivity. With some individuals, these periods of fatigue and hyperactivity seem to be concurrent; in others, one of the conditions will persist for days or even weeks at a time only to be supplanted by the other. These conditions are often seen in children.

Some attribute these symptoms to food allergy or to environmental chemicals. Although this is an attractive hypothesis, there is no evidence that indicates that the syndrome is in fact owing to allergies to food or anything else. There are many people, children and adults, who go through or experience recurring bouts of fatigue and hyperactivity. The symptoms often add up to a problem that interferes with school work, job performance, or family life. It is a serious condition that may require medical attention, attention that may in the end fail to pin down a cause. Nonetheless, there is no evidence at all that any allergic disease, allergic phenomenon, or any component of the immune systems is involved.

Individuals with this syndrome have been targeted by unscrupulous practitioners (physicians as well as a variety of other specialists, legitimate or self-proclaimed) offering exotic, excessive, and usually ineffectual treatments. Be very careful when seeking treatment for this condition.

Depression, Psychosis, and Neurotic Behavior

There are physicians who describe themselves as clinical ecologists. Their practice is founded on the belief that contact with chemicals, preservatives in food, food itself, and its products can significantly affect the nervous system. As we have repeatedly pointed out, what we ingest can affect our behavior. Some foods cause headaches in susceptible persons; specific allergy or sensitivity to certain foods can produce colic, diarrhea, hives, itching, and other allergic reactions. Nonetheless, there is no evidence that food products, chemicals, or preservatives can bring about the psychiatric symptoms—neurosis and depression—that the ecologists say they produce. Although we are not beyond being persuaded that such may be the case, we know of no data to support the belief.

We do know that people exposed to certain toxins, the metal lead, for example, have long been known to develop extensive pathology, including diseases of the nervous system. However, toxins like lead not only have specific behavioral effects that have been cataloged but, more important, their presence can be detected in the body and is reflected in measurable changes in the blood, the bone marrow, and sometimes the kidney. No such observations or measurements have been offered by the clinical ecologists. In the absence of scientific data to support their hypotheses and their therapeutic regimens, we have no enthusiasm for them and recommend that they be avoided.

The Yeast Connection

Another group of physicians assert that a raft of psychological or physical symptoms are owing to the fact that we have become allergic to yeast or Candida. They offer dietary and other treatments, some of them quite bizarre, that are billed as managing the hypothetical generalized invasion of the body by yeast. The alleged yeast connection is based on anecdotal information with very poor documentation. There are no controlled scientific studies to support their musings. However, much like the clinical ecologists, the yeast faddists seem to offer an easy out. We are deeply skeptical of this approach; pursuing it will certainly turn out to be expensive, probably ineffectual, and possibly harmful, especially when it denies your child the benefits of a medically sound approach.

Arthritis

There have been scattered medical reports that arthritis is made worse by certain foods, particularly milk. The Arthritis Foundation has conducted numerous studies of the possible relationship of food to arthritis. It is possible that a small number of people with arthritis show sensitivity to specific foods, but the weight of the evidence indicates that food allergy in and of itself is not a cause of arthritis, nor does food allergy bring on other diseases as well, including irritable bowel syndrome, Crohn's disease, and systemic lupus erythematosus.

Bed-Wetting

There are a number of causes of eneurisis or bed-wetting. Some of them may be serious and organically caused, reflecting problems in the urogenital system. Others are simply a matter of maturity and go away as the child develops. There is no evidence that bed-wetting is related in any way to allergies. There are, however, some allergy medications that increase urine output and make bed-wetting more of a potential problem. One of these is theophylline, a drug commonly used to treat asthma. Theophylline, in addition to dilating the airways and relieving breathing difficulties, stimulates the kidney to make more urine. Since asthmatic children routinely take theophylline at bedtime, it is quite usual for such children to need to urinate during the night. Since children tend to sleep profoundly, the result may be bed-wetting. If this occurs and your child is on theophylline, we think it important for you to discuss the problem with your family doctor or pediatrician and obtain alternative medication.

Dealing with Problems Effectively

One of the best resources to have in dealing with obscure or mysterious symptoms in your child is an understanding and painstaking physician. Too many doctors predicate their practices on writing prescriptions and ordering lab tests. The conditions enumerated above require a great deal of doctor or nurse attention. They use up large bits of time from busy practices, and the fees generated for such evaluations are usually not as high as those that come in from standard procedures and seeing more patients per unit of time. For good physicians who are dedicated to helping their patients, time is not a factor. We have found that one of the most effective ways to deal with problems like these is to help the family understand and to learn to cope with them directly. In so doing, it is amazing how many of these problems gradually fade away.

Understanding and a good measure of hope and optimism about these complaints can often be found in patient encounter groups, parent support groups, or an aggressive program of self-education aimed at understanding and learning to manage the symptoms. Unhappily, all too often parents, understandably beleaguered, look for a quick fix, turning to practitioners who offer overnight cures. This tactic may provide some short-run psychological help, and make child and parent feel better briefly, sustained by the belief that they have found somebody with a magic cure for their problem. Usually the quick-fixed problem comes back, more stubborn than ever on reappearance. We think parents of children with these chronic, troublesome problems should be especially cautious when it comes to choosing a physician, and should read and follow the suggestions in Chapter 22 carefully.

Part Five

Getting the Best, Most Effective Long-Term Care for Your Allergic Child

22

Looking After Your Allergic Child

While health care delivery systems are undergoing a great deal of change, the primary responsibility for the care of your child still rests with you, the parent.

This is particularly true if you are in an HMO or rely, as so many do, on an emergency room or drop-in clinic. Under these conditions, there may be little or no continuity in care. Whether or not there is continuity in medical care you are the very best—perhaps only—person to know what is really happening with your child, and you certainly have the keenest interest and the largest stake in seeing to it that she or he is helped. It is up to you to become educated, and involved in your child's care, to find out what the problem is, its causes, its treatment, and, most important, its prevention. The first step in providing sound care is to find the right doctor.

What to Look for in a Physician

Virtually every family doctor or pediatrician will faithfully carry out routine aspects of care—weighing children in, inquiring about eating habits and school adjustment, discussing physical and social development, treating the occasional rash or fever, and looking after the immunization series advocated by the American Academy of Pediatrics. Much of this care can also be provided by well-trained family nurse practitioners or physician assistants. The key element in the medical care of the majority of children entails learning to recognize the acutely ill child who requires urgent and aggressive treatment, and knowing when and how to use appropriate remedies judiciously.

For children with allergies, the choice of a physician becomes a much different matter. Allergies are likely to persist throughout childhood and well into adolescence, and they sometimes turn out to be a lifelong problem. Children with allergies see their physicians more often, they have more colds and other respiratory infections, and they are quite prone to have multiple allergies, all above and beyond the ordinary problems that other children have. Where an allergic child is involved it is vital that you become intimately involved, both in choosing your child's physician and participating in the ongoing care for the condition. Here are some important matters to consider when choosing a doctor for your allergic child.

1. Do you feel comfortable with your doctor? Is your doctor inclined to be brusque and hurried, or does he/she take time to respond to your questions and concerns fully and understandably? To what extent are you provided with literature on your child's problem? (There are excellent booklets available from groups like the American Academy of Allergy and the American Respiratory Association on allergies and asthma. Your doctor can easily arrange to and should see to it that you have these informational/instructional materials.)

2. Is the doctor a graduate of an accredited American medical school? Although we do not wish anyone to think that there are not outstanding physicians who are graduates of foreign medical schools, standards in American medical schools are quite strict and reasonably uniform. In choosing a graduate of an American medical school, you can be sure that the doctor has met certain minimum criteria of training and competence. (Your local library will be able to direct you to a list of accredited medical schools.)

3. Is your doctor well-trained and board-certified to practice as a family physician, pediatrician, allergist, or other specialist? On graduation from medical school, the new doctor receives a diploma that declares that the recipient can practice medicine and surgery. In truth, this new graduate is not allowed to practice anything. He or she must first pass rigorous written examinations—state or national boards, depending on the part of the country. In addition, graduating physicians must, at the very least, complete one year of postgraduate training known as an internship. Following successful completion of the internship, they are eligible to practice medicine and would once have gone out in the world as general practitioners. In fact, there are very few young general practitioners anymore, since the great majority of physicians recognize the need to take additional training in specialties, such as family practice, internal medicine, pediatrics, surgery, and so forth. These programs require from two to five additional years of study and supervised experience, depending on the specialty. Once this advanced training phase is completed, they take another examination, and if they pass, they become specialists in the area they have chosen.

Thus, family practitioners will have on their walls a certificate testifying that they have passed their board certification by the American Board of Family Practice. Similarly, a pediatrician or internist will display testimony from the American Board of Pediatrics or the American Board of Internal Medicine. Some physicians, a minority, elect to train even further to do work in subspecialties. These may include allergy and immunology, chest diseases, or specialties within surgery like orthopedics. Once again, stiff exams are required at the close of this phase of training.

What this all means is that properly qualified allergists, for instance, should have, at the very least: certification that they have passed the American Board of Internal Medicine or American Board of Pediatrics requirements and documents stating that they have passed and been certified by the American Board of Allergy and Clinical Immunology.

Ask the doctor or nurse about the doctor's specialty and certification status. Get a definite yes or no answer to your question. Do not accept or be misled by the statement that the doctor is "board eligible," but has not yet taken the exam *unless* he or she is a new arrival in the community. Such newcomers are entitled to a period of grace before they have to sit for their exam. Also, do not take your allergic child to other specialists, such as an "Ear, Nose, and Throat" doctor. If you want the best, see a board certified allergist, not a generic substitute.

4. Do not wait to choose a doctor until sickness strikes; make your choice when your child is well. Select a pediatrician, family practitioner, or physician during pregnancy. (HMOs or health plans allow for this type of choice.) Talk to family, friends, and coworkers about likely possibilities. Then, ask for an appointment so that you can check out the doctor while introducing yourself. You will find that virtually everyone will be willing to meet with you and discuss his or her practice and his or her office procedures. This first meeting is a good time to check on training and board certification.

That first visit is also a good time to find out about the cost of visits and attitudes toward treatment. Make especially sure the physician cares about prevention and is not just concerned about treating you or your child when sick. He or she should ask questions about your dietary and health habits. You should be asked about feeding plans or procedures—breast or formula. If your initial visit is with your newborn, the doctor should inquire about weight, eating behavior, sleep patterns, and so on. It should be absolutely clear to you that the doctor puts the highest priority on preventing rather than treating illness.

5. Find out about emergency care. Does your doctor close up shop at 5:00 pm? Who covers during off duty hours? Are you told just to go to the local emergency room or is the doctor associated with a group of physicians that provide regularly staffed acute care coverage after hours and on weekends? To what extent is telephone consultation permitted and encouraged? Can you call your physician for advice rather than having to bring your child in? (Many good physicians reserve an hour during the day for telephone calls and consultation with their patients.) If your doctor is part of an HMO, find out who covers him/her when he or she has gone.

In short, is your doctor ready and willing to provide the kind of help you need whenever it is needed? If so, fine; if not, look elsewhere.

6. Get what you are paying for. Your doctor should allow a minimum of 20 minutes for *any* new examination. This should include a complete and detailed history, including discussion of mother's health during pregnancy, childhood illnesses, family history, and discussion of school attitudes and performance. There should be a complete examination—looking in the eyes and ears and listening to the chest. Where skin problems are concerned, the whole body should be looked at and children must be asked to strip down to their underwear so that no part of the skin goes unobserved. In the case of asthma and hay fever, it should include a detailed examination of the nose and feeling of pulses, right to the extremities, fingers and toes. Where indicated as necessary, it may also include laboratory tests and possibly chest or sinus X-rays.

Choosing a Subspecialist

For children with stubborn and serious allergic problems, such as chronic eczema or moderate to severe asthma, it is important that your child be seen by a specialist. If you can, choose an HMO that facilitates rather than impedes access to a specialist. Although most primary care physicians like pediatricians and family practitioners are well-equipped to take care of mild allergic conditions, we believe that care of chronic conditions requires evaluation and treatment by someone who has specialized training. Consulting a specialist helps to affirm the accuracy of the diagnosis while assuring that you are receiving the most up-to-date treatment, and that treatment will be modified to reflect the development of new therapies or the introduction of new medications.

There are three specialists most often involved in the care of allergic children: allergists, dermatologists, and pediatric chest physicians. Each of these specialists has received the additional training and should display the board certification mentioned earlier in this chapter.

Children who have eczema should see a dermatologist who will usually be someone recommended by your family doctor. However, you ought to observe the same procedures in choosing a dermatologist that you did in choosing your doctor; inquire about board certification and so forth. If you do not feel comfortable with the first person consulted, most communities have a number of dermatologists (the yellow pages of the telephone directory or the local medical society lists these and other specialists), so make another choice.

Deciding between an allergist and a chest physician often is a more difficult decision. For routine allergies that do not involve asthma, one should generally consult an allergist. An allergist should have board certification and should be capable of making the appropriate decisions regarding skin testing, prescribing appropriate medical therapy, and addressing issues of environmental control and preventive measures which are so important to the management of allergies.

As a group, allergists are well-trained and their level of proficiency far better than it was 15 or 20 years ago, before recent and dramatic advances in knowledge in the field. Even so, there is a pitfall that patients who go to some allergists may encounter. These allergists depend economically on the number of skin tests that they conduct. As a result, they carry out more allergy tests than is medically necessary or even advisable. You do not want your child made into a veritable pincushion unless extensive testing is clearly indicated. Chapter 2 covers allergic evaluation. Review it if the question of skin testing comes up, and involve yourself in this decision process. Be warned if the doctor starts the evaluation by bringing out a tray of skin test materials even before taking a detailed history and doing a physical examination. These two preliminary steps can often determine the cause of an allergy without having to resort to skin testing at all.

Severe childhood asthma that requires periodic hospitalization or emergency room treatment should be under the care of a specialist in chest medicine. For one thing, there are some grave causes of asthma in infancy and early childhood. These include cyctic fibrosis and a rare disease known as GER and both of these conditions require skilled, specialized attention. For another, should your child require hospitalization, it is likely that your pediatric chest physician will care for the child during the acute hospitalization phase. Unhappily, there is a shortage of trained pediatric chest specialists; many communities may not have one at all. In that event, children with chronic asthma may be referred to a specialist in adult chest medicine or to an allergist.

Surviving Under Managed Care

Massive changes in methods of delivering health care have occurred in the last several years. The extent of these changes varies significantly depending on where you live. In California, HMOs are close to universal. In the southeastern United States, they are almost unknown in some communities. No matter where you live, though, unless there is a dramatic intervention by the federal government, managed care is the wave of the future.

Simply speaking, an HMO is a new-age health insurance company—with a difference. Unlike earlier insurance companies, most HMOs were developed for profit only. Not-for-profit health insurance organizations are a vanishing breed. The reasons for these changes and their impact on the cost of medicine go beyond the scope of this book. What is important is how the allergy sufferer can survive under managed care.

Managed care's primary motivation is to make money; that gives you, the patient, little room to try to change their rules on health care delivery. In fact, HMOs do not talk about patients or doctors. To the HMO, you are a health care consumer, and the doctor is a provider. The provider and the consumer have contracts with the HMO to have their health care delivered according to the rules and regulations of the HMO. As Dr. Landa Peno, a former medical reviewer for Humana, one of the largest managed care companies in America, testified before Congress in 1993, "medical necessity is a managed care gold mine." These gold mines exist for the HMO because they can readily exclude reimbursement for certain procedures—especially costly ones—and also deny payment for pre-existing medical conditions. Thus, if you move between employers, it is possible that your new HMO will refuse to pay for treatment of a condition that existed prior to your moving to the new job. Oftentimes, they will have a waiting period of up to a year before any coverage cuts in. In other words, if you have high blood pressure when you join a new HMO, you may be responsible for any costs related to this very common condition, including all medications. HMOs tend to exclude expensive procedures like transplantation. In the case of allergists, one of the big problems of HMOs is that they give patients (consumers) access to only the cheaper, and therefore, older and less effective drugs. Costs of other more modern medications would have to be borne by the patient.

Hopefully, your company or employer gives you the right to select your HMOs. In making a choice, here are some factors to be considered.

1. Is reimbursement permitted for pre-existing conditions, including allergies?
2. Who are the doctors who have signed contracts with the HMO?

3. Are you allowed to keep your existing doctor?
4. Does your doctor receive a set fee for seeing you, or does he or she get a bonus for reducing costs? (This is often known as capitation and incentives.)
5. Is your doctor allowed to discuss all treatment options with you or has he or she signed a gag clause?
6. How much will the HMO actually pay if you are put in the hospital? Will it cover all hospital costs?
7. Are you allowed to switch doctors?
8. Can you see a specialist, like an allergist, without authorization or referral? If you require authorization, how long does it take to arrange an appointment?
9. Can you have your prescriptions filled at any pharmacy or only at specific pharmacies?
10. Which hospitals are you allowed to use?
11. What happens in an emergency? Is there 24 hour access, and how are you covered for emergencies?
12. Does the HMO have a list of authorized drugs or medications? What happens if your doctor wants to prescribe a drug that is not on their list?
13. What exactly does your plan cover? Does it include mental illness, obstetrical services, and treatment for allergies?
14. Are there any data available on patient satisfaction surveys of your health plan? How does it stack up with the competition?

These questions are often difficult to find the answers to. There is no obligation for a private company to make their procedures public. Moreover, because HMOs compete with one another in a field very much in flux, mergers and loss of corporate identity and firm history tend to disappear.

Billy has asthma. He is insured through a large HMO in northern California. He was vacationing with his family in Hawaii and became short of breath. He went to the local emergency room for treatment and was hospitalized for three days. Because the emergency room doctors had not notified the HMO that Billy was in the emergency room, the hospitalization costs were not covered. The HMO did cover the cost of the emergency room, but nothing thereafter since preauthorization had not occurred. The family is suing and the family lawyer is quite confident that they will win, but in the meantime, they are out several thousand dollars and it will likely take several years before this case is resolved.

Before choosing any HMO—or any method of health care delivery for that matter— be cautious and be an aggressive consumer. In particular, read, compare, and analyze the contracts of the competing HMOs carefully and critically, and base your final choice on the breadth, cost, and quality of the services offered. Keep in mind that in health care, as in most other matters, the squeaky wheel gets the grease.

Being a Responsible Parent

There have been scores of books written about effective parenting, and we have no intention of summarizing them here. We would simply like to emphasize that for the effective care of your allergic child, you need to develop the skill, knowledge, and resolve to make decisions about your child yourself. You have to learn to be a responsible parent and the child a responsible patient.

When you bring your child to the doctor, make sure that you tell the doctor everything in all the detail you can. So that you do not forget, write down details of symptoms—what, when, where, how much—before you show up for the consultation. Be very clear. Doctors often try to relax you by easing you into a gentle and probably irrelevant conversation. Do not let this divert you. You are there because you and your child have a problem. Discuss it!

Once the reason for the visit is established and treatment decided on, there are a number of questions you should have the answers to. (It helps, in following and evaluating treatment, to write the answers down.)

1. What is the diagnosis?
2. How long will the condition last?
3. What are the drugs that have been prescribed? What are their possible side effects? How long does the doctor think it will take for the drugs to work? How long will my child need to take the drugs? How exactly ought they be administered (how much, when, by what means)?
4. When should I call if treatment does not help?
5. Should I make a follow-up appointment to see the doctor? When?
6. Is the condition serious enough to warrant seeing a specialist or getting a second opinion?
7. Is there anything I should be doing at home to the environment, diet, and so on, to make the symptoms better?
8. How soon will it be before my child can return to school?
9. What should be done about administering medication during the day, at school?

Psychological Aspects of Care for Allergic Children

The popular belief that some forms of allergic disease (asthma and stomach disorders in particular) are psychologically caused is without foundation. Extensive, careful scientific research has been unable to find any causal connection between psychological states and wheezing, for instance. Other equally rigorous studies have failed to demonstrate that psychotherapy in its various forms relieves allergic symptoms.

However, there is a chicken/egg question here; although it is true that anxiety does not produce asthma or eczema symptoms, for example, asthma or eczema can and often do provoke psychological reactions that carry physical consequences that can intensify the ongoing allergic reaction. Children with moderate to severe asthma have to fight for every breath. The experience is terrifying; youngsters having a moderate to severe attack frequently wonder if they are going to last through the night. This fear and the associated struggle for breath cause rapid, shallow breathing—hyperventilation—that triggers further spasms in the smooth muscles that surround the respiratory airways and compromises the breathing even more. Thus, fear and hyperventilation combine in a vicious circle.

Children with eczema or other allergic skin complaints experience intense itching. What do you do with an itch? Scratch it. What happens when you scratch an allergic itch? Usually it gets worse. This upward spiral of intense discomfort is frustrating, depressing, and anxiety-producing. These reactions can affect the vascular system, resulting in increased production of perspiration that, in its turn, aggravates the already agonizing itching.

It is also evident that allergies can be associated with conflict in the family or home setting. Some of these conflicts arise out of resistance of the allergic child to the care regimen being administered by the parents; others are associated with simple disagreements—personality clashes that are brought on or intensified because of a chronic allergic disease. These conflicts can be severe enough to produce the kinds of reactions we have described above. Conflict does not itself cause allergies, but it is capable of setting off physiological reactions that can make them worse.

Thus, through what can be thought of as a kind of feedback loop, an allergic reaction can provoke psychological reactions, which act to intensify the original symptoms. This sort of problem can be managed fairly easily by taking appropriate medication or adopting other tactics (e.g., diaphragmatic breathing or stress-reducing exercises in asthma) that address the primary symptoms. Each of Chapters 10 through 21 contains a section that presents measures that relieve primary allergic symptoms.

Secondary Psychological Effects on Parents

The widely held and erroneous belief that allergies in children stem from psychological causes rooted in malparenting has caused a lot of unnecessary grief. Parents who believe this myth—and there are millions who still do—experience an enormous amount of unnecessary and destructive guilt. They needlessly blame themselves for the troubles their kids are having, and they want to but are unable to figure out what they have done wrong so that they can right matters. This parental guilt is probably the most pervasive and severe consequence of allergic disease and one that is quite unnecessary. The obvious antidote—and one that, unhappily, parents seem to have great difficulty in accepting or applying—is to come to the firm realization that they may have passed on genes that made their kids subject to allergies, but nothing else that they did or did not do caused their child's symptoms.

The task of caring for allergic children also has its psychological fallout. The symptoms themselves can be immensely frightening to the parent; watching an asthmatic child fight to breathe, not knowing quite what to do to help, or having done all that one can without apparent effect is extremely upsetting.

The symptoms that affect the respiratory system or skin almost invariably disturb and disrupt the child's (and parents') sleep patterns, producing stress, frustration, or even anger.

The need to be constantly aware of and vigilant about avoiding or controlling triggers calls for unceasing alertness and, sometimes, a heavy addition to the workload at home. This, too, can heighten tension and cause conflict within the family.

Care for an allergic child can disrupt work, recreation, and other activities; it may create a situation where the parents feel that other, nonallergic children in the family are being deprived of their fair share of care and attention because of the demands of the illness.

Also, the existence of a moderate to severe allergy can so sensitize the parents to the condition that they become unnecessarily and even dangerously overprotective of the ailing child.

These factors can demoralize parents, heighten conflict within the family, and help to set off anxiety or depressive reactions. Allergies, in short, can wreak psychological havoc in the family.

Parents can control damage from the psychological fallout of allergic diseases by applying a combination of knowledge and ameliorative strategies. Here are things you can do to keep your life on an even keel when faced with an allergic child.

1. Understand at the outset that you and your spouse could not have caused the child's symptoms.
2. Learn as much as you can about the disease—what causes it, what you and the child can do to avoid it, to recognize its early warning symptoms, and to treat it. (You will need help from your doctor to do this; *see* the relevant chapters in Part Three of this volume.)
3. To the extent possible, share the information about the nature and cause of the disease with the child. Whenever feasible, have the

child assume at least some level of responsibility for observing avoidance tactics and making treatment decisions.

4. Keep in mind that the child is not to blame for the condition, may be extremely uncomfortable with and frightened by it, and certainly does not want it.

5. Distribute the care of the child as equitably as possible. Both parents, where present, should be directly involved in the care of the ailing child, sharing in all its aspects.

6. Try to avoid becoming overprotective and, in effect, putting a cocoon around the child. Doing that will only add to your labors and stretch out your problems.

7. If interpersonal conflict between any combination of allergic child, parents, and other children erupts, move immediately to work through and resolve the problem as harmoniously as possible.

8. Learn how to recognize and cope with your own stress. There are any number of ways of doing this, from exercise and physical activity to hobbies, to discussing the situation with another person, to biofeedback, to meditation, to counseling or therapy. Sometimes medication, such as tranquilizers, can help, but steer clear of alcohol and beware of becoming chemically dependent.

9. Keep in mind that the symptoms are quite likely to be short-lived, can almost certainly be treated successfully, and probably will not carry any long-term effects.

Secondary Psychological Effects on Children

Children can experience a variety of psychological reactions that may complicate the allergic picture. In some instances, the symptoms will (as we have already seen) carry physiological side effects that act to worsen the allergic reaction. Other possible psychological side reactions include malingering, reactions to medication, feelings of inadequacy or depression, or a disposition to test the limits insofar as medication or treatment are concerned.

Malingering, using the allergic condition to get out of something unpleasant, is fairly often seen.

Mrs. B. notes that her son Keith, now 12, has been complaining that he is having an asthma attack every Tuesday. She is suspicious of this because the symptoms are mild and clear completely by evening. She checks with the school and talks with the principal and Keith's teachers. The physical education instructor mentions that on Tuesdays he brings in a guest teacher who puts the boys and girls through a program of gymnastic exercises that include vaulting, acrobatics, and trampoline work. The instructor goes on to say that Keith obviously dislikes this session, and since he has great difficulty doing some of the stunts, he is teased unmercifully by his classmates. Mrs. B. discusses this problem with Keith, who finally grudgingly admits that his convenient symptoms were largely put on to spare him embarrassment at school.

Where malingering is suspected, the appropriate tactic is to try to find out the reason for the behavior and then to do something about its cause. If there is no apparent reason, then it may be that the home situation is simply more congenial than the alternatives. Where this is the case, a "time out" from positive reinforcement may correct the matter. This entails withdrawing some of the amenities that make staying at home preferable to carrying out other activities—confining the child to room and bed, withdrawing television, radio, hi-fi, video or other games, withholding attention, denying access to telephone, computer, the net, and so on—in short, making the child act in a fashion consistent with the claim of illness.

Reactions to medication often take on psychological overtones. Use of antihistamines, especially, can cause drowsiness and lassitude; other medications can cause jitteriness, hyperactivity, or irritability.

To deal with these drug-related conditions, make sure that you know the potential side effects of any medication your allergic child is taking. If one turns up, contact the physician who prescribed the medication at once and ask for further instructions. For most allergic conditions whose treatments are capable of producing psychological side reactions, there are alternative medications available that (although they may be more costly or more difficult to administer) will not have the youngster in a daze or so hyper that you cannot deal with him or her.

Feelings of inadequacy or depression grow out of some severe, chronic, and stubborn allergic conditions—asthma, skin allergies, and hay fever in particular. Moreover, the simple knowledge that one has to go through an entire life-time watching out for a trigger like food dye or peanut butter is enough to provoke feelings of depression.

Where the feelings can be traced to the disease itself, the child is best helped by being given the opportunity and the support necessary to participate in substitute activities that are satisfying and ego-boosting. For every forbidden pursuit there are literally hundreds of satisfying, challenging and safe alternatives.

Finding acceptable substitutes may take some time and effort, both to narrow down the possibilities and then to get the youngster started. Focusing on the wide array of possibilities—and they are there, even for the most seriously ill child—and helping the child to start and stay with the ones preferred will prove to be rewarding and ego-boosting. Certainly it beats sitting around nursing feelings of inadequacy or depression.

Testing the Limits: Nobody wants to be dependent on medication or to have their activities curtailed for any reason. Individuals with any form of chronic disease are continually tempted to test the limits to see if the underlying condition, possibly controlled by medication or otherwise quiescent, has gone away.

For those with allergic diseases, this temptation is particularly strong, because when the symptoms are controlled or dormant, they are not health-compromised in any way. It is almost as if the disease never happened. So, the individual says, "I think I have got this thing licked," and to test the hypothesis, does something that will put him or her at risk, just to check matters out, to see if the problem is history.

For true allergies, the symptoms may moderate over time, but the potential for an allergic reaction, if the right set of circumstances pops up, is always there. Once allergic, always allergic!

Regardless of what we say we know, people, because of their powerful underlying need to think of themselves as being whole and in control of their destinies, will continue to check to see if they still have their allergies. Since most allergies are mild, usually no harm results from this sort of experimentation. Where a serious, chronic condition is being played with in this way, there may be ugly consequences. We ardently wish that children with these chronic diseases (and their parents) would trust us on this one. The symptoms may not be around right now, they may not be as bad as they once were, and maybe they are not giving as much trouble as they used to. Let well enough alone. Do not find out the hard way that the underlying condition is still lurking, waiting to pounce.

23

Pitfalls to Avoid in Treatment

Ralph, 8, has moderate asthma that usually shows up with a respiratory infection. His condition seriously concerns his mother, who keeps going from one treatment approach to another in the hope of finding a "cure" for Ralph's wheezing. Over the past three years, he has seen a chiropractor, an acupuncturist, and a psychic "healer" as well as the family doctor; he has taken a whole string of home remedies—the one consisting of a steaming hot mug of "natural" honey, lemon juice, and bourbon whiskey made him very sleepy, impaired his breathing, and put him in the emergency room; he has swallowed massive doses of vitamins, minerals, and trace elements; he has briefly followed a succession of "free" diets; and he has eaten more "health" foods than one would believe possible. His symptoms meanwhile just keep going on.

Over the past 15 years a valuable series of studies has focused on the extent of and the reasons for nonadherence to treatment regimens for chronic conditions. These investigations have been extremely revealing. Even for moderate to severe chronic diseases (including allergic complaints), more than half of all patients fail to stick with the course of treatment prescribed by their physicians. Complete or partial nonadherence to what the doctor orders is the rule rather than the exception in patient behavior.

Why is there this massive failure to stick with medical recommendations? There are a number of factors involved that have to do with the complex interrelationships among physician, patient, the nature of the disease itself, and the treatment prescribed.

The Physician

The doctor is often at fault for patient failure to adhere to treatment. Some of the more common ways in which doctors promote nonadherence include failure to explain the nature of the disease or the treatment for it adequately; misdiagnosing the ailment; or prescribing inappropriate treatment. One shocking study revealed that, on the average, doctors spent fewer than 10 minutes treating patients with respiratory conditions. This is simply not enough time to do a competent and thorough examination and history, let alone make a sure diagnosis and explain what may be a complex, multifaceted treatment regimen.

Your responsibility as the parent of an allergic child is to insist, as is your right, that your physician take whatever time is necessary to assess your child's condition thoroughly, to explain the cause, nature, and course of the disease and its treatment in terms you fully understand, to line out strategies for you to follow if treatment proves ineffectual ("If this does not clear up or gets worse in the next 3 or 4 days, call me"), and to recommend consultation if there are any problems or difficulties with either diagnosis or treatment.

The Patient

Patients or their care providers—parents—often have agendas that get in the way of effective treatment of allergic diseases in children. The ways that patients can fail to adhere to treatment are legion; the most prevalent ones include impatience with a slow rate of progress or improvement, over or undermedicating, and "testing the limits."

Any chronic disease makes serious demands on the patience and good judgment of both sick child and parents. The disease wears on, the child improves slightly or not at all, tempers fray, and patience wears thin. The resulting discouragement and frustration prompts parents to look to other sources of aid in finding a cure for the condition. Also, with any chronic disease, allergies included, there is no shortage of alternative treatments— all of them certainly less effective than the up-to-date, advanced medical procedures we have described and many of them potentially hazardous for the patient.

These alternatives hold out one thing in common—hope—false hope, with disappointment being the payoff. Although it is difficult to do, parents should reject the temptation to hop from one treatment to another. Chiropractors, herbalists, homeopaths, psychic "healers," and acupuncturists are not going to cure your child's allergies; mail order medications, home remedies, and various kinds of exotic "tests" advertised in pulp magazines or junk mail flyers ("cytotoxic," hair analysis) will not do it either. The pressure and the temptation to look to other unorthodox forms of treatment are understandable. Resist them. The remedies will turn out to be expensive failures.

Over or undermedicating is another form of nonadherence to prescribed forms of treatment. In some allergic conditions—especially asthma—this can be dangerous. Undermedication happens as much as 80% of the time in children with moderate to severe asthma.

Undermedication is likely to happen when symptoms fade or go into remission; with the child appearing to improve, there is an understandable tendency to cut back on administering medication, which can be a time-consuming, costly, messy, and emotionally taxing activity. Overmedication occurs when symptoms reappear or rebound and stems from the popular fallacy that if a certain amount of medicine is good, more of it is better. Not only is this wrong; in the case of certain medicines used to treat respiratory allergies (theophylline in particular) it can be hazardous or even lethal.

To avoid misuse of medication, parents should be absolutely clear on exactly how much medication their child should have and for how long a period, to be informed about and know what to do in the event of negative side effects, and to know when to return for advice in the event the treatment fails or complications set in.

Related to the preceding points is the all too human tendency to test the limits. Once the allergic symptoms disappear or moderate, most people are tempted to see if they can get along without prescribed medication or to engage in forbidden activities. No one, children included, likes to be dependent on medication; most people do not relish having to think of themselves as limited in some way. They resent having to give up or forgo pleasurable activities out of fear that they will provoke an allergic reaction. "I wonder if I can get along without this darned Theo-dur?" "Just a little helping of this shrimp dip shouldn't hurt me." "The cat looks so lonely and miserable out there in the rain. Letting her in for just a short time shouldn't start me sneezing and wheezing."

Parents and children need to support one another and understand, and accept the feelings of anger and frustration that accompany allergies and their treatment. By listening to one another, being aware of the likelihood of these feelings, and being honest in admitting to them, the temptation to pretend the condition no longer exists is lessened. Where the feelings of anger, frustration, or denial persist, short-term counseling or joining a support group designed to help individuals who have or who are affected by those who have the condition often proves to be a positive step.

Misunderstanding Allergic Disease

Misunderstanding the nature of allergic disease causes difficulty, especially in the case of the chronic, more stubborn forms. In most instances, the normal course is for an allergy to flare up. Treatment is then applied, and the symptoms go away. This spawns a temptation to believe that the condition is gone for good since, ordinarily, there is no residual effect—the child appears completely normal, and there is usually no permanent damage. Gradually safeguards are suspended, and parents are less vigilant and insistent about helping the child to avoid triggers. It is true that most (but not all and not always) childhood allergic or hypersensitive reactions moderate with maturation. This leads parents to the belief that the child has "outgrown" the condition or is free of it. For true allergies, the conditions that caused the original flare-up are always present; they are an ineradicable part of the genetic makeup of the child.

Remission of symptoms should not be taken as evidence of a cure. At best it is a flight into health that with unflagging attention to avoiding triggers, can be prolonged indefinitely. The potential for another reaction, given the right set of circumstances, will accompany the allergic child always.

Another prominent and enormously damaging fable has to do with the cause of allergic disease. At one time it was thought that allergic disease was psychogenic, that is, it was psychologically rooted with something in the individual's emotional life triggering the symptoms. This view prevailed in some scientific-medical circles for a period of about 20 years until the mid-1960s when the role of IgE in allergy and especially the allergic triad of asthma, hay fever, and eczema became absolutely clear and irrefutable. (Individual psychological factors can complicate allergies, as discussed in Chapter 22, but they are *not* the cause.)

Despite the clear repudiation of the unsubstantiated hypothesis that allergies grow out of psychological causes, belief in it has persisted. Even some physicians (and many other uninformed or misinformed health care professionals, including nurses, psychologists, and counselors) hold to it and it is epidemic in the public at large.

There is no persuasive evidence to support the contention that allergies are psychologically caused; treatment strategies founded on this belief will certainly turn out to be costly failures.

The Treatment

The nature of the treatment prescribed is often enough to cause its own downfall. There are a number of prominent reasons for this.

1. *The treatment carries severe side effects.* For allergic diseases, these can range from drowsiness or torpor to severe respiratory or gastrointestinal complications. Physicians should but do not enumerate possible side reactions, nor do they spell out what is to be done if complications turn up. Parents should demand this information; they can also inform themselves easily enough by consulting the *Physician's Desk Reference*, which should be in your local library branch.

2. The treatment is difficult or unpleasant. Many of the medications, especially the ones for respiratory allergies, have an extremely unpleasant taste that impels resistance in children who will give Academy Award quality performances (including sobbing, retch-

ing, breath-holding, and other displays) to avoid taking the drug. Most drugs do come in forms that can be ingested without the child having to taste it; ask the doctor for an alternative form if your child finds the medication difficult to get down.

In addition to unpleasantness, some treatments are abandoned because they are taken improperly and thus do not work. Inhalers are notoriously misused; some researchers have found that they are ineffectively used in three-quarters of cases. (Chapter 11 contains a section telling how to use inhalers correctly.)

In addition, treatment may entail several medications to be taken according to a fixed time schedule and in a definite sequence under specific conditions. You, the parents, should be clear about the schedule and sequence, and see that it is carried out as ordered. If this is not done, the whole process may be useless.

3. *The treatment is tedious, and shows little or no apparent immediate gain.* This is true of some preventive measures like breathing or diaphragm-strengthening exercises for asthma. Children (and adults, too) tire of such routine activities; they can be made more attractive by associating them with other pleasurable activities and by making them as much like a game as possible.

4. *The treatment is essentially preventive in nature.* Medications like cromolyn (for asthma) or nasal steroids (for hay fever) have to be taken in the absence of symptoms or before they are likely to occur. Children who feel well resist taking medication, partly because they see no valid reason for it. The connection needs to be explained to the child and the treatment, despite its apparent needlessness, enforced. Some parents find this authoritarian intervention difficult; if it is a problem for you, ask yourself whether you want a child who is resentful for a short period of time—or one who is sick and miserable.

5. *The treatment is expensive.* Some asthma and hay fever medications, especially, are quite expensive and the mere cost factor is enough of a temptation to have parents cut back on or suspend dosage. This sort of economizing is not only short-lived, but it can have the child developing a serious—and seriously expensive—condition as well.

24

Vaccines, Immunization, and Viruses

Vaccines have virtually wiped out most common childhood diseases. They have done this by helping children (and adults, too) to develop an immunity that protects them from the disease-causing agent.

The general principle of immunization was hit on by Sir William Jenner, a Scots physician, almost 150 years ago. Jenner noticed that milkmaids, women who milked cows, were prone to develop cowpox, a mild skin infection, but almost never contracted smallpox, a deadly disease widely prevalent at that time. Jenner reasoned that cowpox (which the women contracted by coming in contact with the cows' udders) was a weak form of smallpox and that having it somehow made the milkmaids resistant to the killer disease. He then induced cowpox in well people by scratching their skin and introducing an extract from cows' udders into the wound. The result? The people treated in this way developed a mild case of cowpox, but never got smallpox.

Smallpox, once one of the most dreaded of all diseases, was declared eradicated not too long ago; since Jenner's time, vaccines have been developed to confer immunity to diphtheria, measles, mumps, pertussis (whooping cough), poliomyelitis, rubella (German measles), and tetanus. Other vaccines for special at-risk groups are available for tuberculosis, hepatitis, and pneumococcal pneumonia.

These pneumococcal pneumonia vaccines have been marvelously effective. In this country, the combined number of reported cases of all these diseases has declined, in the past half-century, from over one million to fewer than 10,000 per annum.

How Immunization Works

Immunization entails either stimulating the body to manufacture its own disease-fighting antibodies—active immunization—or administering preformed antibodies that confer temporary immunity—passive immunization. In the case of active immunization, a vaccine or toxoid is introduced into the recipient's body. (Vaccines contain killed or weakened organisms that cause the disease; toxoids carry bacteria that have been made nontoxic, that is, they cannot trigger the disease, but they have the ability to stimulate the body to produce its own antitoxins or antibodies.) Preformed antibodies that confer passive immunity are usually derived from serum (blood), either human or animal.

In general, vaccines made from live, weakened microorganisms confer lifelong protection, and the immunization needs only be done once; in other forms of vaccines, booster shots may be required periodically.

Immunization and Your Child

Providing your child with a proper series of immunizations is a vital ingredient in his or her health care; most states in the United States have laws that require school children to show evidence of vaccination before they are first enrolled. However, because allergic diseases are linked to or are the outgrowth of immunological disorders, immunization presents special risks for allergic children that need to be taken into account. You and your doctor should weigh the undoubted advantages of immunization procedures against the heightened risks they pose for some allergic children. Here is a summary of the vaccines employed for various diseases, their usual side effects, and a discussion of any special problems or contraindications they represent for allergic youngsters.

Diphtheria, Tetanus, Pertussis (DTP)

When and for Whom? The combined DTP vaccination is routinely recommended for all normal infants and children. It is usually given as a series of five injections according to the following schedule:

Age	Immunization Number
2 months	1
4 months	2
6 months	3
18 months	4
4 to 6 years	5

Tetanus boosters alone are then recommended every 10 years or so; the first of these would be given at about age 14 to 16.

Usual Side Effects of DTP: Each of the three components in the DTP vaccine has its own unique profile. The diphtheria vaccine is generally innocuous; few if any significant reactions to it have ever been reported. Tetanus, however, can cause significant local tenderness with muscle aches and pains around the site of the injection.

Of the three elements in DTP vaccine, the major offender is pertussis. Pertussis can produce swelling and pain at the injection site. Rarely, it can also lead to fever, convulsions, and even death. Pertussis vaccine has succeeded in virtually eliminating whooping cough in much of the world; it is an important and powerful public health tool. However, the pain and swelling their children experience is more than some parents want their children to endure. We suggest you discuss this with your physician. Generally, we recommend routine use of pertussis vaccine in normal children unless earlier reactions to the vaccines have been particularly troublesome.

DTP for Allergic Children: Pertussis has a side effect that has been demonstrated experimentally; when animals are given the pertussis vaccine, they often produce more of the IgE antibodies that can generate allergies. Children who are atopic (*see* Chapter 1, pages 7 to 8) and already have a high incidence of allergies make far more IgE than they need. Thus, following administration of pertussis vaccine, their allergies may grow significantly worse. For this reason, we do not recommend pertussis vaccination in any child who has a history of moderate to severe hay fever, asthma, or eczema.

Effectiveness of DTP: The DTP vaccine is remarkably effective. These diseases have all but disappeared from our population; when outbreaks of them occur, they are almost always found only in children who have not been immunized.

Measles, Mumps, Rubella (MMR)

When and for Whom? Containing live but weakened or attenuated viruses, MMR is administered as a combined vaccine. It is usually given at 15 months of age as a single, one-time immunization. The body makes an immune response to the weakened virus, which then protects against the real virus. The weakened virus is enough to induce an immune response, but it is not enough to cause significant disease. We recommend MMR for all normal children.

Usual Side Effects of MMR: Live virus vaccines contain small numbers of the "bugs" that must divide and multiply in the body to induce the immune response. Therefore, reactions to all three of these live virus vaccines are fairly common. Measles provides a good general example. In a significant number of children, mild fever and a slight rash *may* occur about 5 to 12 days following immunization.

MMR for Allergic Children: MMR may be contraindicated if your child reacts to materials used in the laboratory to make the product. These materials may include egg proteins and/or antibiotics. For this reason, it is important that you let your doctor know if your child has any sensitivity to egg whites or antibiotics.

Additionally, since a live virus is being administered, it is absolutely imperative that your child have normal immune function. Children whose immune systems are compromised—those born without a normal immune system, for example—may not be able to kill the attenuated viruses. This deficiency may even prove fatal. Most physicians are acutely aware of this possibility, and such immune-compromised children are usually treated so gingerly that virtually all parents of these children know of the risk. However, they may not be aware that the live virus can be spread from a normal child to a child with the compromised immune system.

> Jeb has had reduced immune function all of his life from a rare disease known as DiGeorge syndrome. He was born without a completely normal thymus. He received a thymus transplant at birth and has done fairly well, although he is still very susceptible to infections. When he was three years of age, his sister, Helen, received her measles shot at 15 months as recommended. Helen did fine, but about a week later, Jeb began to show signs of severe, disseminated measles.

Effectiveness of MMR: MMR has also been oustandingly effective. In the United States in 1949 there were over one million cases of measles, mumps, and rubella combined; in 1985 the total came to just over 6000.

Poliomyelitis

When and for Whom? Polio immunization has generally been conferred through administration of an oral vaccine that contains weakened strains of polio virus types 1, 2, and 3. The viruses remain in the mouth, moving eventually to the gut, and are finally excreted in the feces. The presence of the viruses in the gut is enough for the body to make a sufficient antibody response to safeguard the child. Recently, however, the American Academy of Pediatrics has recommended the use of two injectable doses in addition to oral vaccine. Consult your child's doctor for the latest information. We recommend completion of the polio vaccine series.

Usual Side Effects of Polio Vaccine: Polio vaccine almost never carries side effects; on extremely rare occasions, the virus can mutate and become disease-causing again. This is an unlikely event, so rare it is best disregarded.

Polio Vaccine for Allergic Children: We urge polio vaccination for all except immunity-impaired children. In their cases, it is also well to note that the live virus is carried in the stool; children with compromised immune function can receive the virus by coming in contact with the feces of other children or adults.

Effectiveness of Polio Vaccine: In 1952, the peak year for polio in the United States, 21,269 cases were reported; today polio is rare.

Other Vaccines

Influenza: Influenza vaccines (flu shots) are relatively effective, although the form or type of the virus changes from year to year so that the vaccines given may not be specific to what is going around this year. The usual side effects are soreness and fever. Rarely, the vaccine may trigger Guillain-Barre syndrome, a progressive, but reversible nerve paralysis that starts in the feet and ascends up the body.

There are no contraindications of flu shots for allergic children. Although their effectiveness is open to some question, if influenza does develop in an asthmatic child, its consequences can be quite serious, making the asthma much worse. On balance, we advocate flu shots for asthmatic children; the potential benefits far outweigh the potential risks.

Pneumococcus: Pneumococcus vaccine protects against the bacteria that cause pneumonia. Most children have good immune systems and ward off this disease readily; even if it does develop, it responds quickly to antibiotics. Accordingly, the vaccine is not called for in most children, normal or allergic. However, children who have had their spleens removed or children with sickle cell anemia should receive this vaccine because their ability to combat pneumonia bacteria is impaired. (Sickle cell anemia is a blood disease found primarily in ethnic groups who have migrated to the United States from areas where malaria is endemic: Africa, the Mediterranean rim, and Central America.)

Hepatitis: There are three major types of hepatitis (liver) infections—A, B, and C. Hepatitis A, the most common form, is generally spread by fecal contamination of foods. It is most often encountered in crowded, unsanitary living conditions, but it is relatively benign, of short duration, and has no significant side effects. Hepatitis A can be guarded against most effectively by observing good hygiene habits and avoiding foods susceptibile to fecal contamination (seafoods, especially shellfish and certain other foods, depending on locale).

Gamma-globulin, an extract from blood of healthy individuals who carry hepatitis A antibodies, also provides limited immunity. If you plan on traveling to Central America, Asia, or Africa, the new hepatitis A vaccine provides excellent protection.

Hepatitis B, serum hepatitis, is a much more serious and stubborn disease. Sometimes fatal, it can cause extensive liver damage. It is most often spread through use or sharing of contaminated hypodermic needles, syringes, or through blood transfusions; it is frequently encountered in intravenous drug users; it can also be transmitted sexually. The risk of contracting hepatitis B by ordinary individuals is slight and vaccination for it is not routinely indicated. There is a hepatitis B vaccine available for use by

individuals in high-risk groups—physicians and other health care providers.
Hepatitis C is a serious infection transmitted by contaminated blood products. There is no vaccine.

Smallpox

Smallpox was declared eradicated a few years ago, and smallpox vaccinations are no longer routinely given to children. Even so, the disease represents something of a danger, because (in order to guard our armed forces from the threat of biological warfare) all members of the military continue to receive smallpox vaccinations. As a result, every year there are a few instances of newly vaccinated persons carrying the weakened virus home where children whose immune systems are deficient in some way come into contact with and contract the disease. Even more common is the spread of the virus to children with eczema. Skin with eczema is *very* susceptible to the virus in the vaccine, and death may even occur! Therefore, ironically, the only real threat from this once virulent killer grows out of the vaccination procedures that did away with it. The danger is, of course, miniscule, but if you are in the military and have a child with an impaired immune system or eczema, you should be aware of the remote possibility of the virus being passed on or if your immunity-compromised child is in contact with military personnel or their children, you should check out the situation with your physician.

There are other vaccines not in widespread use and not ordinarily given to children: plague, yellow fever, cholera, typhoid fever, tuberculosis, Rocky Mountain spotted fever, rabies. For children, allergic or not, there are no special circumstances associated with these vaccines except that some of them are prepared or cultivated by using eggs. Here again, if your child is allergic to eggs, administration of one of the egg-grown vaccines could trigger a reaction. Alert your doctor to this possible complication as you work to achieve an optimal level of immunity in your children.

AIDS and Your Child

The acquired immune deficiency syndrome (AIDS), epidemic is in its 15th year. At its outset in the United States, it struck primarily young, homosexual males; today the disease plays no favorites, affecting people of all ages, ethnicities, and conditions—including children. Most youngsters are infected when the AIDS virus is passed on to them by their mothers during pregnancy. The virus travels from the infected mother, through the placenta, to the unborn child. The child then harbors the virus and is born infected. We discuss the syndrome here because the effects of the virus are to compromise—shut down—the immune system, just as the name given the disease suggests.

Recent surveys have indicated that up to 25% of newborn children in some areas of major cities test positive for HIV, the AIDS-causing virus. The infected child, after a latent period that lasts anywhere from months to years, then develops the symptoms, which can include recurrent infections, diarrhea, and failure of the child to grow or prosper.

Although the newborns make up the largest contingent of child-aged sufferers, growing numbers of adolescents are turning up with the disease. Intravenous drug users and individuals who neglect to follow safe sexual practices are particularly susceptible to infection.

Children with AIDS, despite their compromised immune systems, do not develop allergies at a rate different from that seen in the general population. Asthma, particularly asthma associated with respiratory causes, does turn up, and for the most part, since AIDS victims have limited life expectancies, they display the type seen most often in young children—viral-induced bronchospasm.

Children with the human immunodeficiency virus (HIV), the cause of AIDS, who also have asthma are treated in much the same way as other asthmatic children with one major exception. While beta-agonists are prescribed to dilate the airways, Intal or Tilade are administered to combat inflammation, and inhalants are taken as needed. Steroids do not come into use. Steroids, as noted elsewhere in this book, heighten the risk of infections and impair local immunity. Because youngsters with HIV are already more susceptible to pulmonary, nasal, and sinus infections, introducing steroids to the treatment mix can render the child terribly vulnerable to infection.

Another troublesome problem for children with AIDS and their care providers has to do with the problem of diagnosing asthma. Pulmonary infections and AIDS go together, and because of this pairing, the presence of asthma in the child can go undetected and untreated.

Also, there are other wrenching problems with AIDS-infected children: They are often cruelly and callously ostracized, closed off from human contact and interaction because the general public still does not understand that it is virtually impossible in ordinary contact for the disease to go from an affected child to one clear of symptoms. This plague mentality persists in the face of both fact and reason. Furthermore, they are much more likely to have little or no access to medical treatment of any quality whatsoever, and home care is at best skimpy for the most part, given the fact that the mother herself has the virus or the disease, or may already be dead.

Neonates with HIV had no part in the process that led to their infection. They are truly innocent victims. School-age children are a different matter. They can and should learn to take steps that will protect them from contracting this tragic disease. They need to be educated about the disease itself, what it is, and how it is transmitted. In particular, they need to be aware of the dangers of using illicit intravenous drugs—heroin, cocaine, and methamphetamines in particular. They also need to know the dangers of promiscuous and unprotected sexual activity.

Parents represent the first line of defense for these youngsters. They can and should get the facts about AIDS and transmit them to their children. They should monitor their children's behavior, attitudes, and associations, and talk openly with them about problems or questions they have about how and with whom their offspring are spending time. Limits need to be settled on and enforced—going out to the park at 10 o'clock on a school night, for example, spells nothing but trouble.

Beyond that, parents should realize that there are helping resources in the school and community, and be prepared to use them if the need—or the suspicion of need—arises. Schools do offer AIDS awareness courses. School counselors are trained to work with children who are at risk or in trouble. Community organizations, churches, and other entities sponsor programs that encourage and provide opportunities for children to spend their time constructively, and in ways that are rewarding and beneficial.

Also, parents not only need to monitor, guide, and instruct, but they also need to remember that they are forever cast as models and that their own behavior sends signals to their offspring. The joint-smoking parent who gets after the child for experimenting with marijuana lacks credibility—and brains for that matter.

A Special Note on Gamma-Globulin

Gamma-globulin is the antibody-containing fraction of donor blood that is often useful in preventing infections. Children without the ability to make antibodies can be given shots once per month containing antibodies derived from healthy people. These shots are often enough to permit them to lead a normal life; without them the child would die.

> Doug is an 11 year-old with Bruton's syndrome. He was born without the ability to make antibodies. His younger brother, Steve, also had this disease. (It tends to run in males.) Before Doug was diagnosed as having Bruton's syndrome at age 18 months, he had recurrent bouts of pneumonia and ear infections. His doctor finally did a total serum antibody test and found that Doug had a major reduction in the normal antibody level. He has been receiving an injection of gamma-globulin every month since the discovery and has been virtually symptom-free.

Gamma-globulin has been used primarily in children like Doug who have congenital immune deficiency diseases. In fact, a major improvement in the use of gamma-globulin has followed the recent introduction of an intravenous preparation that is delivered directly into the blood of the recipient rather than by intramuscular injection, as was done formerly. The new preparation has fewer side effects and seems to work much better at preventing infections.

Gamma-globulin can also be used as a prophylactic in individuals who have been or are likely to be exposed to certain diseases—hepatitis A especially. If you or your children plan on traveling to a high-risk hepatitis area, it is often routinely recommended that you and they receive a hepatitis-preventive injection of gamma-globulin. The passive immunity that the injection confers by putting somebody else's antibodies to work will protect against hepatitis.

Ironically, the major side effect of gamma-globulin is allergic reactions. Because you are receiving injections of protein from someone else, you may make antibodies against it, and this can result in swelling, fever, and enlargement of lymph nodes and spleen. It can even trigger an acute anaphylactic or shock reaction. If you have never experienced them before, it is unlikely that they would occur, but the possibility of such a reaction does exist.

Gamma-globulin shots are extremely expensive, so they are not likely to be given routinely and are not recommended except under the special circumstances mentioned above.

A Special Word for Expectant Mothers

Live virus vaccinations are *never* recommended for women who are trying to become or are pregnant; any vaccination at all during pregnancy should be discussed with your physician. The use of such vaccines, especially rubella (German measles), can significantly damage the fetus.

It is routinely recommended that all women of child-bearing age receive a blood test to see if they are immune to rubella. If they are not, then rubella vaccination should be administered at a time well in advance of any planned pregnancy. Exposure to the attenuated rubella vaccine is just as injurious to the fetus as if the mother actually caught German measles.

Information on Vaccines

Information on vaccines can be obtained by calling your local Department of Public Health or by writing or calling:

Division of Immunization
Centers for Disease Control
1600 Clifton Road, NE
Atlanta, GA 30329
(404) 639-3311

A Note on the Needle

Vaccinations and other injections are immediately and sometimes sharply painful, and children quickly learn to associate this abrupt pain with visits to the doctor's office. When the child is told of an upcoming visit to the doctor, fear, dread, and even hysterical crying before and during the event can occur.

You can make things easier for your child and the doctor by taking some simple precautionary steps.

1. Do not emphasize the fact that there may be a vaccination or injection.
2. *Never* use the threat of injection as a means of enforcing discipline at home. (It is surprising how many parents tell their children that if they do not behave, they will be taken to the doctor for a shot.)
3. If there is to be a shot, let the child know shortly in advance of the event that it will be given and why; let the child make any possible decisions about where the injection is to be made and to share in the process to the fullest extent possible.
4. Treat injections as the ordinary, run-of-the-mill events they are. Reinforce cooperative or unafraid behavior; help get rid of rebellious reactions or tantrums by reminding the child that the pain and discomfort were short-lived, and commending cooperative behavior.
5. Let the doctor know in advance if the child reacts strongly against injections so that he or she can be prepared. If you know strategies that keep your child relatively calm or quiescent, let the doctor know what they are and advise their use.

Getting the child to the point where he or she accepts injections (and blood drawing) as routine aspects of medical care carries a number of important advantages for parents, physician, and child.

For allergic children, asthmatics, and those with eczema, in particular, the intense emotional reaction to the needle in some youngsters can provoke or intensify symptoms. In other children where a serious conditioned fear reaction is present, the actual injection or the mere sight of the needle can bring about a vascular collapse with dizziness, fainting, or even more severe consequences.

Allergy Shots

A special type of vaccine is the injection of extracts prepared from allergens into patients. This is commonly known as allergy shots or immunotherapy. The only people who should receive allergy shots are those who clearly have IgE-mediated disease as revealed by skin tests and a clear history. In most instances, your physician can predict by the history whether the symptoms justify the allergy shots or not. Just because you have positive skin tests does not mean that you would be helped by shots.

The allergy shots are done by preparing a dilute mixture of the allergens you are allergic to. Thereafter, once or twice a week, you will receive an injection in your arm. With each visit, and assuming you have not had a bad reaction, the dose—its strength or concentratedness—of the shot is increased. Following each injection, you must stay in the doctor's office for at least 30 minutes in case you show signs of a local or a systemic reaction. A local reaction can be as mild as some warmth at the injection site or as severe as very bad swelling and pain. A systemic reaction can include shortness of breath, wheezing, hives, and even shock. It is for these reasons that your doctor will observe you for 30 minutes. If a mild reaction develops, the doctor is likely to decrease the dose of shots before proceeding to higher strengths.

The major reason for shots are allergies to the common environmental agents, such as house dust and pollens. Sometimes injections of molds are given, but the data on this approach are poor and often not recommended until further research is done. Allergy shots to counteract sensitivity to pets is only recommended when individuals must be exposed to animals, such as veterinarians. Families who insist on allergy injections in preference to giving up their pets are sometimes accommodated, but the injections are risky, expensive, prolonged, and frequently ineffectual.

Chapters 11 to 15 discuss the relative role of allergy shots in specific problems with children. In general, the major indications would be allergic asthma that is not entirely controlled by pharmacotherapy and airborne allergies that mediate hay fever and allergic conjunctivitis. As noted above, we never recommend allergy shots for patients with eczema, and it is very rare to manage hives with shots. By way of contrast, patients who have life-threatening allergies to insect stings are often very well controlled by injection of insect venom. Finally, we do not recommend the use of allergy shots for food allergy.

25

The Long Haul: What Happens to Children with Allergies?

Thirty years ago, if a child had an allergy, he or she was pretty much stuck with it. Hay fever sufferers could sometimes be desensitized by going through a course of shots of dubious efficacy; persons having severe breathing problems brought on by an acute asthma attack could be helped temporarily by being injected with epinephrine. Then, in all likelihood, they would be referred to a psychiatrist. Effective medications to prevent or control the outbreak of allergic symptoms were all but unknown.

Since that time, immense strides have been made in understanding the mechanisms of allergic disease, and as a corollary to that understanding, various kinds of medications have appeared. We now have an impressive and effective array of allergy drugs—antihistamines, steroids, inhalants, and medications—that combat or forestall symptoms.

Even so, the underlying mechanisms of allergic or hypersensitive reactions are still not well or completely understood. As the biophysiology and biochemistry of allergic reactions come to be more fully known, as they certainly shall, and distinctions between the various forms of allergic disease become more clear-cut, even greater progress will be made in developing strategies and remedies that will allow easy management of these diseases.

Along with the improved medical management of symptoms, the ability to avoid or control allergy-causing substances has advanced greatly. Labeling requirements oblige manufacturers to tell us what processed foods contain, thus providing information that permits allergy-prone individuals to avoid some possible sources of trouble. There are still wide areas that need attention, of course; "fresh" foods, fruit, and vegetables, are, in many instances, not required to carry labels naming preservatives, insecticides, herbicides, or fungicides with which they have been treated or are often contaminated—for instance, sulfites as preservatives on fresh fruits and vegetables were outlawed in January 1987; however, the ban does not extend to potatoes or seafood and the Environmental Protection Agency allows sulfites on fresh grapes provided 40% of the bunches carry warning labels. Users naturally assume that the unlabeled bunches are sulfite-free. Likewise, meats, poultry, fish, and shellfish packages are not obliged to list the preservatives, dyes, or antibiotics that may have invaded them.

As knowledge and concern over the extent to which chemicals have invaded our lives mounts, the supply of goods that has been produced with the intent of avoiding chemical contamination also grows. The chemical threat to health and well-being is being countered to a modest extent by the increased availability of contaminant-free products.

Along with more precise information about what causes allergies and the development of effective medications to treat them, there has been impressive improvement in the efficacy of devices to control the environment. The ability to control air temperature and purity efficiently has been a boon to many allergy sufferers.

There has also been a surge in self-management of symptoms. This move in the direction of self-care has heightened awareness of allergic symptoms and their triggers, and promises to make their management more judicious and effective.

These developments all argue that allergies, although they will continue to be shown by a significant proportion of all children, are likely to decline in significance in years to come. There will be just as many allergic children in coming generations, but with the growth in knowledge about the nature of allergic diseases and the radically improved means of treating them, the symptoms will not be as severe, persistent, debilitating, and costly as they are today.

That is the long haul. What is the outlook for children who have allergic diseases right now?

First, even under today's conditions, the long-term outlook for most children with allergic diseases is quite favorable. What happens during the process of maturation has a great deal to do with that bright prospect. Asthma and eczema usually moderate as the child grows older and continue to be a problem into adulthood in only a small minority of cases. Gastrointestinal difficulties also mostly disappear as the digestive apparatus matures. Hives are inclined to be much more prevalent in youngsters, although the reason for this is not clearly understood.

Hay fever and allergic contact dermatitis are exceptions to the general rule that allergies ease off with age. Both hay fever and allergic contact dermatitis require a period of sensitization before they show. Once the child is sensitized, the symptoms are likely to persist and to become worse over time, but the good news here is that there are extremely effective preventive medications to combat hay fever, and allergic contact dermatitis can be readily controlled by keeping away from whatever it is that triggers the rash.

Growing up helps to lighten allergic symptoms; it also eases some of the nonallergic difficulties brought on by allergies. Chronic earache or eye problems usually abate by the time the child reaches 6 years of age.

Not only will the symptoms usually gradually fade away, but when they vanish, they will carry their signs with them. Asthmatics will not suffer permanent lung damage. The skin recovers, unblemished, from eczema, hives, or contact dermatitis. Most children are likely to escape completely physically unscathed from their allergic experiences.

This should not encourage you to believe that allergies amount to nothing more than a passing nuisance. For many—perhaps most—children they are, but for some kids, they add up to considerably more than that. In a small percentage of instances, the condition, especially asthma or acute sensitivity reactions to things like food or food additives, antibiotics, or insect stings or bites can be life-threatening. Also, the incidence of asthma-related deaths in children is rising. Studies of the phenomenon indicate that the reasons for the increase are complex and many-faceted, but simple disregard of the symptoms, undermedication, and psychological depression are prominent factors associated with asthma-caused deaths. Significantly, all of these factors are more closely tied to the home than hospital or clinic.

Some children do carry their allergies into adult life. Hay fever and allergic contact dermatitis, as noted, are likely to have lifelong runs; asthma, eczema, and hives can also persist for a life-time. Even so, when they do tag along into adulthood, the symptoms can usually be managed by observing a few precautions and sticking with prescribed medication. Most allergic adults are able to get along with reasonable comfort and without having awkward limits put on the range or level of their activities.

Among the potentially most damaging consequences of allergic disease is the psychological impact it can exert on the child. Throughout the book, we have paid a lot of attention to the importance of having the child lead a life as close as possible to normal and have suggested how the allergic child can be helped to do this. This heavy emphasis results from our experience in seeing how often allergies lead parents to shield the child, not only from the consequences of allergy, but from many of the good, enjoyable, fun parts of growing up. Such overprotection can have substantial and long-lasting effects on the child's personality and attitudes, undermining independence and self-reliance, creating dependency and a negative self-image. Although it is true that there may be risks involved in having some allergic children participate in some aspects of the usual run of childhood activities, parents all too often lose sight of the fact that denying the child those experiences carries its own set of potential problems.

In summary, then, the long-range prognosis for your allergic child is upbeat. The chances are good that the symptoms will either be outgrown, or if they do persist, they will probably be avoidable or manageable, even under today's conditions, and will certainly be more so as the nature of allergic disease and hyperreactivity comes to be more fully revealed in the next few years.

As the parent of an allergic child, you can best help in his or her development by trying to see to it that the youngster:

Has knowledgeable, competent, understanding care;

Participates fully and freely in as many of the ordinary aspects of growing up as can be managed; and

Is treated matter-of-factly, and is not allowed to let the disease become an excuse or an occasion for stunting his or her physical, psychological, or social development.

Appendix A

An Elimination Diet

Eat and drink only the foods listed below. All fruits and vegetables, except lettuce, must be cooked, or canned.

Grains and cereals
    Rice
    Rice wafers
    Puffed rice, Rice flakes, Rice Krispies

Fruits
    Apricots
    Cranberries
    Peaches
    Pears

Meat
    Lamb

Beverage
    Water

Vegetables
    Beets
    Carrots
    Chard
    Lettuce
    Oyster plant
    Sweet potato

Oils and seasoning

Olive oil, Crisco, Spry

Any vegetable oil (except oleo margarine)

Acetic acid vinegar (white)

Salt

Sugar (cane and beet)

Vanilla extract (synthetic)

Dessert

Tapioca

Suggested Menu:

Breakfast	**Lunch**	**Dinner**
Rice Krispies	Lamb chop	Lamb patty
Rice wafers	Sweet potato	Boiled rice
Peaches	Beets	Carrots
Apricot juice	Rice wafers	Lettuce with white
Peach jam	Cranberry juice	vinegar
Water	Pears	Peaches
		Apricot juice

AVOID: Coffee, tea, Coca-Cola and other soft drinks, chewing gum, and all medications except those ordered by a doctor.

INSTRUCTIONS: Stay on the basic diet for 14 days. If there are no changes in symptoms, stop the diet, but if the diet seems to be working:

- On day 15 add yellow vegetables all by themselves.
- On day 22 add green vegetables all by themselves.
- On day 31 add chicken all by itself.

Continue adding food groups one at a time at seven-day intervals. Keep a written record of what foods are added, when they are added, and the reaction, if any, to them. Add foods in large amounts, and eat them several times a day during addition period. If a reaction does occur, drop the newly added food or food group, return to the preceding week's diet, stay with it for a seven-day period, and then reintroduce the food or food group associated with the reaction. If the reaction reappears, you have identified one cause or agent. Eliminate that food from the diet and continue adding foods as before until the process is completed.

Appendix B

Food Groupings

1. Apple—apple, pear, quince
2. Aster—lettuce, chicory, endive, escarole, artichoke, dandelion, sunflower seeds.
3. Beet—beet, spinach, chard
4. Blueberry—blueberry, huckleberry, cranberry
5. Buckwheat—buckwheat, rhubarb, garden sorrel
6. Cashew—cashew, pistachio, mango
7. Chocolate—chocolate (cocoa), cola
8. Citrus—orange, lemon, grapefruit, lime, tangerine, kumquat, citron
9. Fungus—mushroom, yeast
10. Ginger—ginger, cardamom, turmeric
11. Gooseberry—gooseberry, currant
12. Grain (cereal or grass)—wheat, corn, rice, oats, barley, rye. Also wild rice, cane, millet, sorghum, bamboo shoots
13. Laurel—avocado, cinnamon, bay leaves, sassafras
14. Mallow—cottonseed, okra
15. Melon (gourd) watermelon, cucumber, cantaloupe, pumpkin, squash, other melons
16. Mint—mint, peppermint, spearmint, thyme, sage, basil, savory, rosemary, catnip
17. Mustard—mustard, turnip, radish, horseradish, watercress, cabbage, sauerkraut, Chinese cabbage, broccoli, cauliflower, brussels sprouts, collards, kale, kohlrabi, rutabaga
18. Myrtle—allspice, guava, clove pimento (not pimiento)
19. Onion—onion, garlic, asparagus, chives, leeks, sarsaparilla
20. Palm—coconut, date
21. Parsley—parsley, carrot, parsnip, celery, celeriac, anise, dill, fennel, angelica, celery seed, cumin, coriander, caraway

22. Pea (legume or clover)—peas (green, field, black-eyed), peanuts, beans (navy, lima, pinto, string, soy, an so on), licorice, acacia, tragacanth
23. Plum—plum, cherry, peach, apricot, nectarine, almond
24. Potato—potato, tomato, eggplant, green pepper, red pepper, chili pepper, paprika, cayenne
25. Rose—strawberry, raspberry, blackberry, dewberry, loganberry, youngberry, boysenberry
26. Walnut—English walnut, black walnut, pecan, hickory nut, butternut

Appendix C-1

Milk-Free Diet

Eliminate:

    Milk, including low-fat, skim, and buttermilk

    Dairy products, including:

        Butter

        Ice cream and sherbet

        All cheeses

        Yogurt

        Cottage cheese

        Sour cream

    Common foods that contain dairy products, such as,

        Puddings

        Custards

        Cream soups

        Breads

        Pastry

        Spaghetti

    All foods that contain (read labels):

        Nonfat dry milk solids

        Sodium (Na) caseinate

        Whey

        Chocolate, cocoa

Appendix C-2

Cereal-Free Diet

Foods Allowed:

Starches
  Tapioca
  White potato
  Sweet potato or yam
  Soybean potato bread
  Lima bean potato bread
  Soybean milk
Meats
  Lamb
  Beef
  Chicken, fryers, roasters
  Capon (no hens)
  Bacon
  Liver (lamb)
Vegetables and fruits
  Artichoke
  Asparagus

Beets
Carrots
Chard
Lettuce
Lima beans
Peas
Spinach
Squash
String beans
Tomato
Apricot
Grapefruit[a]
Lemon
Peaches
Pineapple
Prunes
Pears

*Preservatives, flavorings, food
preparation aids, and so forth*
  Sugar, cane or beet
  Salt
  Sesame oil
  Soybean oil
  Willow Run oleomargarine
  Gelatin (Knox's), flavored
    with allowed fruits and
    juices
  Maple syrup or syrup made
    with cane sugar flavored
    with maple
  White vinegar
  Vanilla extract
  Lemon extract
  Corn-free baking powder
  Baking soda
  Cream of tartar

[a]The canned fruits should be preserved with cane sugar, not corn sugar. Water-packed fruits may be used and sweetened with cane sugar syrup.

Appendix D-1

Tyramine-Free Diet

Eliminate:

Chocolate, cocoa, fava beans

All ripened cheeses

Avocados

Bananas

Canned figs

Fermented sausage (e.g.,
  bologna, salami, pepperoni,
  aged beef, hot dogs)

Red wine, sherry

Beer

Chicken livers

Pickled herring

Anchovies

Dried fish

Yeast extracts

Appendix D-2

Salicylate-Free Diet

Eliminate:
1. Foods
   Almonds
   Apples
   Apricots
   Blackberries
   Cherries
   Cucumbers and pickles
   Currants
   Gooseberries

   Grapes and raisins
   Nectarines
   Oranges
   Peaches
   Plums and prunes
   Raspberries
   Strawberries
   Tomatoes

2. Flavorings (artificially flavored and colored foods and drinks)
   Breakfast cereals with artificial
      coloring and flavoring
   Ice cream
   Oleomargarine
   Cake mixes
   Bakery goods (except plain bread)
   Jello (gelatin)

   Licorice
   Mint flavors
   Oil of wintergreen
   Jams and jellies
   Lunch meats (salami,
      bologna, etc.)
   Hot dogs

3. Beverages
   Cider and cider vinegars
   Wine and wine vinegars
   Soda pop (all soft drinks)
   Diet drinks and supplements
   Gin and all distilled drinks
   (except vodka) and
   similar beverages

   Kool-Aid
   All tea
   Beer

4. Drugs and miscellaneous

    All medicines containing aspirin, such as Bufferin, Anacin,
        Excedrin, Alka-Seltzer, Empirin, Darvon compounds, and so forth
    Perfumes
    Lozenges
    Mouthwash
    Toothpaste and toothpowder (baking soda can be used as a substitute)
    Note: Check all labels of prepared foods and drugs for artificial
    flavorings or coloring.

Foods allowed:

1. All meats (except those that are artificially flavored, such as hot dogs, bologna, and so on)
2. All fish (except fish sticks)
3. Eggs
4. Milk and milk products
5. Butter or Willow Run margarine (purchase at health food stores)
6. All vegetables (except cucumbers and tomatoes)
7. All starches—plain bread, rice, potato, pancake mixes without coloring
8. Fruit—grapefruit, lemons, pears, bananas, dates, limes, figs
9. Beverages—coffee and Seven-Up
10. Others—pure maple syrup, all vegetable oils, distilled white vinegar, salt and pepper

Note: Tylenol may be used for fever or pain (purchase at a pharmacy).

Appendix D-3

Mold-Free Diet

Eliminate:

All cheeses, including cottage cheese, sour cream, sour milk buttermilk

Beer and wine

Cider and homemade root beer

Mushrooms

Soy sauce

Canned tomatoes, unless homemade

Pickled and smoked fish and meats, including sausages, hot dogs, corned beef, pastrami, pickled tongue

Vinegar and vinegar-containing foods, such as mayonnaise, pickles, pickled vegetables, green olives, sauerkraut

Soured breads (e.g., pumpernickel), fresh rolls, coffee cakes, other foods made with large amounts of yeast

All dried and candied fruits including raisins, apricots, dates, prunes, figs

Melons, especially cantaloupe

Appendix D-4

Foods and Other Materials Containing Tartrazine

Tartrazine is a dye (FD&C yellow #5) added to foods to "improve" their appearance. The list below is only suggestive of the literally thousands of places it may turn up. Read labels carefully. A typical label may read as follows: "INGREDIENTS: Enriched wheat flour . . . whole wheat flour... oil shortening... sugar, corn syrup, salt, malted barley flour, lecithin, FD&C yellow #5, and artificial color."

Baked goods, bread with food
   dyes added, sweet breads,
   wheat

Butter

Candies

Cereals, colored

Cheeses

Chips (potato, corn, taco)

Fish, frozen (some; check label)

Fruits, canned (some; check label)

Ice creams

Jello (gelatin)

Lozenges

Margarine

Meats, prepared

Mouthwash

Mustard

Pudding

Sauces and gravies, prepared

Toothpaste

Yogurt

Appendix D-5

Foods and Other Materials Containing Sulfiting Agents

Metabisulfite (sodium bisulfite) is a food preservative and freshener. It is commonly used to keep prepared potatoes white (beware of fast-food french fries) and, until recently, was sprinkled on trays of ingredients at salad bars to maintain their appearance of freshness. It also turns up in many processed foods and beverages, including beer and wine. Here is a typical label for a product containing metabisulfite. "INGREDIENTS: Cauliflower, vinegar, salt, dill, alum, and sodium bisulfite."

Beer

Cheeses

Cider

Cordials

Fruit juices

Glucose (syrup and solid)

Jello (gelatin)

Pickles

Potatoes, whole, peeled, or sliced (raw)

Sausages and sausage meat

Vegetables, dehydrated

Vinegar

Wines (red, white, or rose)

Appendix E

Pollen Map and Guide for the United States[a]

Map area	Trees[b]	Grasses[c]	Weeds[d]
CT, ME, MA, NH, NJ, NY, PA, RI, VT	Maple/Box Elder Oak Birch	Timothy Orchard Fescue Redtop	Lamb's-quarter Ragweed, giant and short Cocklebur
DE, DC, MD, NC, VA	Maple/Box Elder Birch Juniper/Cedar	Redtop Vernal grass Bermuda grass Orchard grass Timothy	Pigweed Lamb's-quarter Ragweed, giant and short Mexican fire bush
II FL (North), GA, SC	Maple/Box Elder Birch Juniper/Cedar	Redtop Vernal grass Bermuda grass Orchard grass Rye grass	Lamb's-quarter Ragweed, giant and short Sagebrush English plantain
V FL (South)	Box Elder Oak Juniper/Cedar	Redtop Bermuda grass Salt grass Bahia grass	Pigweed Lamb's-quarter Ragweed, giant and short Sagebrush
V IN, KY, OH, TN, WV	Maple/Box Elder Birch Oak Hickory	Redtop Bermuda grass Orchard grass Fescue Rye grass	Waterhemp Pigweed Lamb's-quarter Ragweed, giant and short
VI AL, AR, LA, MI	Maple/Box Elder Juniper/Cedar Oak	Redtop Bermuda grass Orchard grass Rye grass Timothy	Carelessweed/Pigweed Lamb's-quarter Ragweed, giant and short

(continued)

Map area	Trees[b]	Grasses[c]	Weeds[d]
VII MI, MN, WI	Maple/Box Elder Alder Birch Oak	Redtop Brome Orchard grass Fescue Rye grass	Waterhemp Lamb's-quarter Russian thistle Ragweed, giant and short
VIII IL, IA, MO	Maple/Box Elder Birch Oak Hickory	Redtop Bermuda grass Orchard grass Rye grass Timothy	Pigweed Lamb's-quarter Mexican fire bush Russian thistle Ragweed, giant and short
IX KA, NB, ND, SD	Maple/Box Elder Alder Birch Hazelnut Oak	Quack grass/ Wheat grass Redtop Brome Orchard grass Rye grass	Waterhemp Pigweed Lamb's-quarter Mexican fire bush Russian thistle Ragweed, false, giant, short and western
X OK, TX	Box Elder Juniper/Cedar Oak Mesquite Orchard grass	Quack grass/ Wheat grass Redtop Bermuda grass	Waterhemp Carelessweed/Pigweed Saltbush/Scale Lamb's-quarter
XI AZ, CO, ID, MT, NM, UT, WY	Box Elder Alder Birch Juniper/Cedar Oak	Quack grass/ Wheat grass Redtop Brome Bermuda grass Orchard grass	Waterhemp Pigweed Saltbush/Scale Sugarbeet Lamb's-quarter Mexican fire bush
XII AZ (Desert), CA (Southeastern Desert)	Cypress Juniper/Cedar Mesquite Ash Olive	Brome Bermuda grass Salt grass Rye grass Canary grass June grass	Carelessweed Iodine bush Saltbush/Scale Lamb's-quarter Russian thistle Ragweed, false, slender, and western
XIII CA (Southern coastal)	Box Elder Cypress Oak Walnut Acacia	Oats Brome Bermuda grass Orchard grass Salt grass	Carelessweed/Pigweed Saltbush/Scale Lamb's-quarter Russian thistle Ragweed, false, slender, and western
XIV CA (Central valley)	Box Elder Alder Birch Cypress Oak Pecan	Redtop Oats Brome Bermuda grass Rye grass Orchard grass	Pigweed Saltbush/Scale Sugarbeet Lamb's-quarter Russian thistle Ragweed, false, slender, and western

(continued)

Map area	Trees[b]	Grasses[c]	Weeds[d]

XV
  ID (Southern),
  NE
	Box Elder
	Alder
	Birch
	Juniper/Cedar
	Ash
		Quack grass/
		  Wheat grass
		Redtop
		Brome
		Bermuda grass
		Orchard grass
			Pigweed
			Iodine bush
			Saltbush/Scale
			Lamb's-quarter
			Mexican fire bush
			Russian thistle

XVI
  OR (Central
  & Eastern),
  WA (Central
  & Eastern)
	Box Elder
	Alder
	Birch
	Oak
	Walnut
	Pine
		Quack grass/
		  Wheat grass
		Redtop
		Vernal grass
		Brome
		Orchard grass
			Pigweed
			Saltbush/Scale
			Lamb's-quarter
			Mexican fire bush
			Russian thistle
			Ragweed, false, giant,
			  short and western

XVII
  CA (North-
  western),
  WA (Western),
  OR (Western)
	Box Elder
	Alder
	Birch
	Hazelnut
	Oak
	Walnut
	Ash
		Bent grass
		Vernal grass
		Oats
		Brome
		Bermuda grass
		Orchard grass
		Salt grass
			Pigweed
			Saltbush/Scale
			Lamb's-quarter
			Russian thistle
			Ragweed, false, giant,
			  short and western

ALASKA	Alder Aspen Birch Cedar Hemlock	Blue grass/ June grass Brome Canary grass Fescue	Bullrush Dock/Sorrel Lamb's-quarter Nettle Plantain
HAWAII	Acacia Beefwood Juniper/Cedar Cypress	Bermuda grass Corn Finger grass Johnson grass Love grass	Cocklebur Plantain Kochia Pigweed Ragweed, slender

[a]Only the more common and widespread pollens for each area are listed.
[b]Pollenating season ordinarily late winter through spring.
[c]Pollenating season ordinarily spring through early summer.
[d]Pollenating season ordinarily summer through early fall.

This botanical region map of the United States is reproduced with permission of Miles Pharmaceutical Division, West Haven, CT. It is reproduced from Botanical Regions of the United States and Canada, 1975.

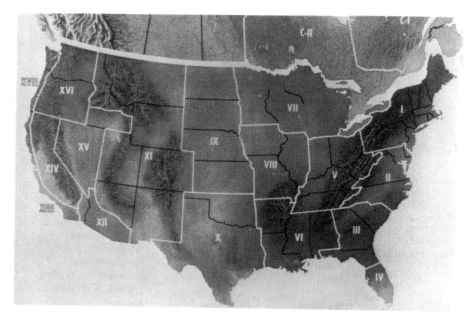

Pollen map and guide for the United States.

Appendix F

Where to Find Allergy-Relieving Products

Catering to the needs of allergy sufferers has become something of a growth industry, fueled by the spiraling incidence and severity of allergic diseases. Suppliers of materials, devices, and services aimed at avoiding or controlling exposure to triggers of allergic disease are no farther away than your telephone.

There are two excellent general lists of sources. The first is *The Asthma Resources Directory*, a comprehensive compendium of thousands of products, services, and resources for allergy problems. The directory costs $29.95 and is available from the Allergy and Asthma Network, 3554 Chain Bridge Road, Suite 200, Fairfax, VA 22030-2709, 1-800-878-4403.

Also useful is the *Allergy Products Directory*, a somewhat more modest publication that may be ordered from the Allergy Publications Group, P.O. Box 640, Menlo Park, CA 94026-0640. It costs $9.95.

Most localities have suppliers of needed materials and supplies. Depending on your needs, you may find what you are looking for under the following headings in the phone directory's Yellow Pages.

Air Cleaning and Purifying Equipment

Air Conditioners

Air Conditioning Equipment and Systems—Repairing

Clean Room—Installation and Equipment

Dust and Fume Collecting Systems

Dust Control Materials

Environmental and Ecological Services

Health Appliances

Health and Diet Foods—Retail

Hospital Equipment and Supplies

Safety Equipment

Water Filtration and Purification Equipment

Water Softening and Conditioning Equipment—Service and Supplies

The Health and Well-Being, Home Interior and Decorating, and House Remodeling and Garden Indexes of the "smart" Yellow Pages will also provide leads. Actually it is probably best to start with your own physician, HMO, or allergist by asking them to suggest local sources of supply and, where indicated, to issue you a prescription for what you need. (When prescribed by a physician, most insurers will defray the cost of equipment and supplies.)

Index

233

About the Authors

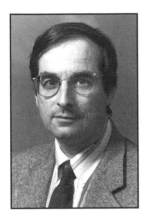

Dr. Gershwin is the holder of the Jack and Donald Chia Endowed Chair of Medicine at the University of California at Davis School of Medicine. He graduated summa cum laude from Syracuse University with a major in zoology and received his medical degree from the Stanford University School of Medicine. Dr. Gershwin received his training in internal medicine at Tufts University and in immunology at the National Institutes of Health. He is a former Guggenheim Fellow and has been Chief of the Division of Allergy, Rheumatology, and Clinical Immunology at the University of California since 1982. Dr. Gershwin has authored 15 books and more than 400 experimental research papers. He has received numerous honors and has lectured at more than 100 Universities throughout the world.

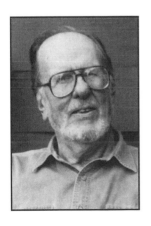

Edwin L. Klingelhofer earned his PhD in psychology at the State University of Iowa in 1953. Since 1977, he has worked as a free-lance writer, publishing technical and popular articles on a variety of subjects as well as short fiction and cinema and play reviews. He has also authored or co-authored five books during that period, three of which, in collaboration with Dr. M. Eric Gershwin, are on allergy-related topics. He resides in Sacramento, California with his wife of 52 years, Jean.

Dr. Gershwin and Dr. Klingelhofer have written many books and articles, both as a team and individually. Together they wrote the much praised *Living Allergy Free* (Humana, 1992). Dr. Gershwin is editor of *Diseases of the Sinuses* (Humana, 1996).

Dr. Klingelhofer is author of *Coping with Your Grown Children* (Humana, 1989).